"Hillary and Brad Keeney have written an amazing book! It exceeds the promises in Gregory Bateson's writing. When therapists discovered cybernetics, many started using its vocabulary without living up to its promises—not the Keeneys. *Circular Therapeutics* transcends that disconnect and offers compelling accounts of what cybernetics can do when actually embodied in practices of living, not merely talked about. It opposes following therapeutic theories and advocates instead surrendering one's preconceptions to an involvement in the kind of virtuous circularities that can bring forth learning, healing, and improvisation—not just for clients but, in the evenhanded spirit of cybernetics, for therapists as well. *Circular Therapeutics* boldly challenges the therapeutic profession with the wisdom of an interactive poetics that evokes creative involvement. I recommend it to anyone who is open to constructive ideas, whether they are therapists willing to overcome their entrapment in the theories of traditional schools, ordinary folks ready to engage in healing communications within their communities, and even cyberneticians as it teaches everyone a lesson in its offering of a circular way of being in communication with one another."

—Klaus Krippendorff, Ph.D.
Gregory Bateson Professor for Cybernetics, Language, and Culture, The Annenberg School for Communication
University of Pennsylvania

"*Circular Therapeutics* invites us into a dance of helping, healing, learning and knowing. While focusing on helping relationships, Hillary and Brad Keeney offer us profound insights into the very systemic ideas that are at the heart of being human. As such, it is a book that should be read by therapists, cyberneticians, and systems thinkers, but also dancers and poets. And it is a book where we, as readers, become engaged with the wisdom of improvisational performance. It is a sheer delight that inspires positive movement in many senses; movement in our thought, movement in our bodies; with ourselves; and with others in a joint improvisation."

—Frederick Steier, Ph.D.
Professor of Communication, University of South Florida, and Former President, American Society for Cybernetics

"I honor and celebrate the way the Keeneys are asking therapists to open their hearts to healing ways! Their work is a wonderful teaching and blessing."
—Flordemayo
Traditional healer, Founding Director, Institute for Natural and Traditional Medicine, member of the International Council of Thirteen Indigenous Grandmothers

"This fantastic book is a much needed contribution capable of transforming the entire thinking and practice of therapy! Our profession is headed toward 'scientific delirium madness' if we do not embrace what the Keeneys tell us about finding the healing heart of therapy. They teach us how to bring transformational creative magic—authentic mojo—into every therapy session. Bravo!"
—Stephen R. Lankton, LCSW, DAHB
Editor-in-Chief of the *American Journal of Clinical Hypnosis* and author of clinical books including *The Answer Within, Practical Magic,* and *Tools of Intention.*

Circular Therapeutics
GIVING THERAPY A HEALING HEART

Circular Therapeutics

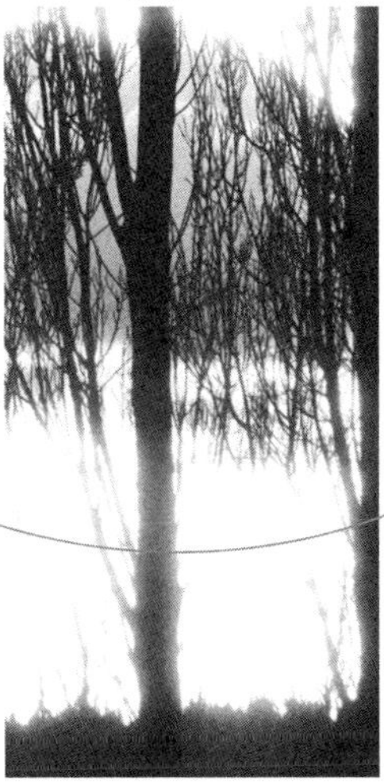

GIVING THERAPY A HEALING HEART

Hillary Keeney
with Bradford Keeney

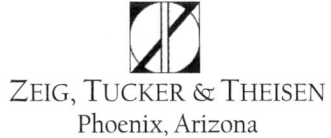

ZEIG, TUCKER & THEISEN
Phoenix, Arizona

Copyright 2012
Hillary Keeney & Bradford Keeney

All rights reserved under International and Pan-American Copyright Conventions. No part of this book may be reproduced, stored in a retrieval system or transmitted in any form by an electronic, mechanical, photocopying, recording means or otherwise, without prior written permission of the authors.

Library of Congress Cataloging-in-Publication Data

Circular therapeutics: giving therapy a healing heart

/ Keeney, Hillary, with Bradford Keeney. — 1st edition.

p.   cm.

Includes bibliographic references and index.
ISBN 978-1-934442-43-2 (alk. paper)
1. Family Therapy   2. Social Systems-Therapeutic use
3. Bateson, Gregory   4. Cybernetics
I. Kenney, Hillary   II. Title

RC480.55.B77. 2012

Published by

ZEIG, TUCKER & THEISEN, INC.
3618 North 24th Street
Phoenix, AZ 85016

Manufactured in the United States of America

DEDICATION

For my mother, Catherine.
With all my love, Hillary

CONTENTS

Foreword xi
1. Giving Therapy a Healing Heart 1
    Interlude 13
2. Deleting Narrative: Purging the Internal and External Chatter 15
    Case Example: The Light Man 42
    Interlude 46
3. Entering Interactivity: Steps To an Embodied Circularity 47
    Case Example: Selling a Cancer 66
    Interlude 76
4. Holding Interactivity: A Batesonian Tool Kit 77
    Case Example: The Green Light 94
    Interlude 104
5. Circular Poetics: Cybernetic Metalogues and Zen Koans 105
    Case Example: Singing to a Lonely Chili Pepper 121
    Interlude 124
6. Clinical Tuning: A Healing Heart Voices Rhapsodic Expression 125
    Case Example: Handling the Family Silver 134
    Interlude 139
7. Circular Therapeutics: Going to the Crossroads 147
    Case Example: Staring at 2,000 Degrees of Fire 158
    Interlude 165

8. The Woman Who Married Jerusalem 167
9. The Weird Family 181
10. Seeing a Ghost 197
11. The Water that Changed Color 209
    Interlude 223
12. On Not Not-Knowing 225
    Interlude 226
13. Koan: Should Therapy Be an Archive or a Beehive? 229
    Metalogue on the Case 230
14. An Invitation 237

References 239

Foreword

Circular Therapeutics is a magical book written by authentic traditional healers who have impeccable scholarship. Hillary and Bradford Keeney have the gift of helping people change. This book is unique in that it aims to heal other therapists and mental health workers who suffer from being overattached to the limiting assumptions, habits, and models their professions prescribe. The Keeneys take on a next to impossible though absolutely critical job of demonstrating how clients and therapists are stuck in the same existential dilemma. Both believe that explanation and narrative direct living, and that suffering is appeased once we discover the best story line or grandest understanding. As practically every long-standing wisdom tradition holds, this kind of knowing removes us from being inside the heart of transformation and the soul of exuberant, creative living. The Keeneys help us grasp what Milton Erickson meant when he insisted that insight is the greatest obstacle to change.

In this book you find a multitiered juggling of the whole human enterprise that is concerned with the compassionate handling of suffering. On one layer, we are reminded of what healing looks, sounds, feels, tastes, and smells like. Interspersed case examples clearly demonstrate and sing the truth that the old art of traditional healing is still alive and kicking in modern times. In addition to bringing us inside the real-time art of performed therapeutic healing, the Keeneys next present a therapy of therapy, an exquisite invitation for therapists to find their healing heart. Here they liberate therapy by first drawing the distinction between interactivity and narrativity, the former pointing to experience itself while the latter nods to all our chitchat about it. Like Zen roshis engaging the reader in mondo, the Keeneys take on the challenge of unshackling the narratives, models, and theories that hold therapists back from being more fully inside the flow or Tao of interaction, the realm of experience less restrained by pre-formed imposition.

Their exorcism of narrative imprisonment draws upon what arguably may be the most content-free conceptual apparatus of our time—cybernetics, the postmodern science of complexity that addresses the patterns that organize events with little concern for the nature or substance of the events themselves. The patterns that relevantly connect are circular and feed upon themselves, like the medieval Ouroborous, the dragon that chases and devours its own tail. In this re-circulation of pattern is found the emergence of those qualities that make us human, the circularities of self-reference, paradox, and autonomy, and all the other themes that have been the subject of cybernetic luminaries from Warren McCulloch to Norbert Wiener, Gregory Bateson, Heinz von Foerster, Francisco Varela, and Humberto Maturana, among others—many of whom I had the privilege to personally know and report on during my career as a reporter of science.

In this one-of-a-kind book, we are taken to the core of cybernetics' most central idea—circularity. There we are turned around for inside the circular patterns that organize organization, we find life freed from that narrator whose name is sometimes called "ego" or "self." At the same time, we find that the achievement of this freedom from compulsive narration has the cost of riding the Ouroborean Ferris wheel. But to get on with our life, we need to get off that carnival ride as well. It is at this level of understanding that our authors offer a healing of cybernetics, first making it analogous to the process of improvisation, and then releasing it altogether. They use cybernetics to get rid of other forms of explanatory story and follow up with the encore of disposing cybernetics itself, doing so for cybernetic reasons—allowing it to devour its own *tale*. One of their intellectual mentors, Heinz von Foerster, did the same and their circular handling of his lineage of thinking would most certainly bring a smile to his face. They accomplish this work with real cybernetic chops, having an excellent grasp of this scholarly tradition, while allowing it to feed back and correct its own tendency to become a fixed narration rather than an ever-turning process of change.

Be warned that the constant motion inside this text may at first seem to bring on a bit of motion sickness. Hopefully you will recognize that this is the fluttering of emotion that is ready for more motion in your practice. Hold on to your desire to be set free from all that gets in the way of your becoming a therapist with a healing heart. Circular therapeutics is a medicine that treats top-heavy therapists who haven't yet become light enough for creative flights in their sessions. I invite you to get on board its fantastic transformative ride for it can carry you somewhere—a journey straight to the circular circus (*circulus*) of virtuous change.

Be aware that you are holding a three-ring circus in your hands. In the first ring, notice how clients may be transformed inside the interactive dance of healing. In the second ring, attend to how therapists may change their ways of changing others by letting go of their habituated models. In the third ring, notice the vehicle that helps therapists cross the stream do its job and then watch it disappear as well. As you move from a model of therapy to being a transformed therapist, watch everything vanish, from therapy to cybernetics. In this disappearing act, we are reminded again and again that we are being offered a poetics of living, a circular therapeutics that invites healing of all dissociations between the ongoing flux of living and our fixed stories about it. Finally, be prepared to experience how the healing heart of therapy is none other than the koan of Zen, the plunge into the life-stream you are already in, but have to cross in order to re-enter.

Listen for the change in yourself as you move through the pages of this book. Watch your inner light flicker as it reveals another way of seeing. Or as the Keeneys might say, feel this book grab hold of you and pull you into God's pot where it can cook you. Anything less leaves you undone.

It may take you years to learn how to live without explanations. Like an extraordinary painting, invent a life that escapes meaning. Change yourself as the means of participating in the change of others, doing so in ways that beg for explanations while defying them. Become an explanation- and narrative-challenged healer. Do so to silence the noise so you may hear the beat of your own drumming heart.

—Paul Trachtman,
former Science Editor of *Smithsonian Magazine*

1. Giving Therapy a Healing Heart

If you needed help handling your own existential suffering and had the choice, would you see the Buddha or a licensed therapist? Similarly, if you wanted to learn how to be a more authentic, transformative presence with your clients, would you choose to hang out with Our Lady of Guadalupe or a best-selling psychotherapy author? Finally, what if you rubbed Aladdin's lamp and a genie came out and asked, "I can give you healing wisdom or therapeutic technique. Which one do you choose?"

Assume that you had previously heard that your colleague met the same genie and had chosen healing wisdom, only to be surprised when the genie replied, "Here's some technique. Master it in order to gain wisdom." Further assume that another colleague with more experience with genies had chosen therapeutic technique. She was not prepared for the genie's training program that taught her how to rub the lamp in a way that brought a giggle to the magical being. Though this uncommon action changed her clinical practice, she still doesn't understand why it works.

Given this background information, let's imagine that you decide to go all the way outside the box of choices and proceed to rub the lamp with exceptional enthusiasm. To your surprise, you spontaneously start singing the genie a song, doing so as if it was the last moment of your life. You are so totally absorbed in this exuberant performance that you close your eyes and sing with all your heart. Tears of joy flow down your cheeks before you start laughing, for you have never felt this alive in all your days. Then you smell a sweet fragrance and open your eyes. To your surprise you have become the genie.

There you are inside a large lamp that is the size of your clinical office. In front of you a client is rubbing his forehead, hoping you will be able to offer some direction for his life. That's the moment you realize that the genie in the lamp has always been the inborn therapeutic genius inside your heart, the deepest source of inspiration, guidance, and creativity that is waiting to come out and help others feel the magic of being alive. But here's the rub: knowing this doesn't help your genie come forth. You must make the right motion, feel the purest emotion, and make some creative commotion in order for it to rise from the caverns of your heart.

We invite you to become a wisdom-based therapist with a healing heart. This cannot be solely derived from technique, nor can mere absence of technique necessarily help. Wisdom cannot be imparted in any systematic way so as to be memorized, rehearsed, and easily replicated. Nothing can be shown or taught in a rational, straightforward way that will automatically help you move from being a licensed mental health practitioner to a shining lamp of healing wisdom.

In the juxtaposition of healing wisdom and therapeutic technique is found something more important than the difference between them. At this intersection, call it the healer's crossroads, we must surrender our habituated, choice-making ways and allow our heart to rise higher than the deliberations and decisions of routine mind. Here an awakened heart sets the stage for creative transformation. Finding the healing heart of therapeutic change begins when we reach the dead end where schooled ways of making a purposeful delivery of therapy are no longer viable.

Healing has a long history, and we sometimes forget that therapy is the youngest established folk healing practice of them all. Taking a more encompassing historical look at the mental health professions—psychotherapy, family therapy, brief therapy, coaching, hypnosis, social work, psychiatry, counseling, self-help psychology, and the like—all the contemporary orientations to people-helping are a relatively new form of profession. Charcot practiced hypnosis in 1870, Freud began psychoanalysis in 1886, Carl Rogers published his major work on client-centered therapy in 1951, followed by B. F. Skinner's call for behavioral therapy in 1953. The 1950s, '60s and '70s led to a proliferation of the major orientations of psychotherapy practiced today. Subsequent therapies were largely recycled forms of earlier distinctions. Suffice it to say that what a licensed therapist knows today is derived from methods of treatment largely developed in the last 60 years.

Now consider the oldest living culture in the world, the Kalahari Bushmen (San) of southern Africa. They have been around for 60,000 years, or longer, and their ancient rock art images depict a form of healing that is thousands of years old. They began creating rock art around 27,000 years ago, and the earliest depictions of healing show the original ways of handling human suffering and sickness. Other indigenous healing cultures also thrived around the world as they developed ways of healing that are thousands of years old. In other words, there has been a whole lot of healing going on in every corner of the globe.

From the larger historical view, we are newborn infants, recent arrivals to the healing scene. Might we benefit from giving more respect to our elders, turning to the ancient healing custodians and asking them to help us learn to walk, run, and possibly fly away from our overly rational, reductionist ways of knowing? Might an expansion of the context that holds therapy help us become more open to diverse choices, strategies, and resources?

Consider whether it is possible that our existential know-how has decreased and devolved as science and technical knowledge have developed. Does wisdom mature with age while gadgets and gadget-like thinking break down easily, waiting for the next new-fangled contraption to replace it? Would you rather have your personal suffering be doctored by someone steeped in deep wisdom or handled by someone whose training prepared him or her to pass a multiple-choice quiz in order to get a union card? Again, given the choice between having a session with the Buddha (or Jesus, Teresa of Avila, Hildegard of Bingen) or a licensed therapist, whom would you choose? Whose lamp holds transformative light?

Our profession has strayed away from the great wisdom traditions and is creatively withering inside the restrictive medical and scientific models where simple statistical measurements determine what form of treatment should be administered to all the challenges of living. What would a panel of wisdom experts say about this? Imagine giving a panel consisting of timeless wisdom keepers – including Confucius, Socrates, Jane Austen and Martha Graham—the opportunity to address the proponents of evidence based models of therapy. Or even fantasize a panel of historical wisdom keepers from our own profession. Consider Milton Erickson, Carl Whitaker, Virginia Satir, Fritz Perls, Carl Jung, Frieda Fromm-Reichman, among others, being asked to evaluate the way therapy is evaluated today. Is the highest good being served or are we choking opportunities for complex communication, creativity, wisdom, and healing to be welcome in clinical practice?

This book is an antidote to the measure-obsessed fundamentalism that claims that therapy is primarily legitimized by simple numerical outcome studies. We do not have to solely answer to the gods of statistics and the legalized drug lords anymore than poets and clergy should have to answer to focus groups and commercial television. We assert that therapy, with its intended purpose of handling and easing human suffering, is a member of the transformative healing arts. Furthermore, wisdom-based therapies are the most experientially potent, holding a complexity that basic measurement cannot assess and simple theory can never explain. Our young folk-healing tradition needs a journey home, a return to the heart of healing that waits to renew our relationship with unlimited possibilities for helping others change.

We are not the first practitioners to recognize the limitations of modern therapy and wonder whether other diverse and more ancient healing traditions might have something to teach us about transformation. However, this book warns against any trivial partnership between therapy and New Age spirituality, appropriated forms of shamanism, generalized iterations of

"Eastern" philosophy, or other spiritual or religious orientations. We must avoid extracting elements of these traditions from their more encompassing contexts and placing them inside the same scientific, psychological, and interpretive premises operating in therapy. We call for *epistemological* diversity rather than a diversity of cultural offerings held inside one way of knowing.

No single culture or healing tradition exclusively holds all the answers to human suffering, and likewise all healing traditions are arguably equal in shortcomings. Consider also that sometimes healers from different cultures find they have more in common with one another than they do with people in their own village. A common characteristic among the great healers and wisdom teachers we have met has been the vastness and immensity with which they can hold all manner of difference, as well as more encompassing patterns of connection. They are able to hold contradictions in practice and thought, are open to change as they are moved by the circumstances of each situation they work in, and reject any theory, model, or orientation that fences them in. Wisdom serves change, complexity, and the paradoxes embedded within processes of transformation. A therapist with a healing heart is a wisdom-based practitioner who is free to shift whenever a process of change calls them to do so.

It ultimately doesn't matter whether your heart awakens with the help of the sound of a meditation bell, a gospel hymn, a jazz standard, or an African drum. Maybe a memory of your grandmother's cooking or the words of a Shakespearean sonnet are what plug you into the greater mystery. If breathing deeply before a session helps remind you that the key to easing human suffering lies deeper than the topsoil of a licensing exam, then by all means tap into the Great Silence of a Japanese *zendo*. But there is no need to build a therapeutic model out of it. Doing so might kill whatever wisdom or vastness the contemplative traditions hold.

Let's not deflate the wisdom of wisdom traditions by squeezing them into a therapy box. And let's not deflate healing by squeezing it into a single, preferred wisdom tradition. Setting the genie free means jumping out of all constructed boxes that separate "therapy" from "healing" from "spirit" from "art" from "music" from "dance" from "wisdom" from "body" from "mind" from "East" from "West". There is a greater dance that never stops weaving the tapestry of transformation. It has given birth to the diverse expressions of healing throughout the world, and it defies the reductive simplicity imposed upon it by our rigid categorizations.

We want to share what we have learned from our own journeys into the ancient wisdom traditions and their healing ways. Brad, who has written numerous classic texts in psychotherapy and the transformative arts, once took a sabbatical from a university teaching position to teach in southern Africa. There he met the Kalahari Bushmen and continued his professorial leave of absence for over a decade as he went on to learn from traditional healers all over the world. Along the way, he became a practicing member of several healing cultures including that of the Bushmen *n/om kxaosi*, the world's oldest form of traditional healing.

Hillary, with a background in social justice work, diversity education, coaching, and community-based leadership development, spent several years studying Zen Buddhism, which included residency at the Zen Center of Los Angeles. She later served as a Frederick P. Lenz Residential Fellow for the study of American Buddhism at Naropa University. As a salsa dancer in Los Angeles and a poet teaching gender studies, multiculturalism, and creative transformation in the university, she later joined Brad to create a traditional healing practice in New Orleans.

This book aims to help connect therapy to the collective wisdom embodied in traditional healing. It cannot be emphasized enough that therapy has operated without meaningful relationship to other healing ways and is too easily seduced by overly simplistic explanations of human experience. Let this be clearly said: there is more to our experiential life than psychology, sociology, introjected objects, externalized problems, and disturbed molecules. When we ignore the unexplainable awe-inspiring mysteries of the complexities sometimes metaphorically referred to as the "divine," we risk losing our connection to the source of what inspires other wisdom traditions to heal one another.

Have the mental health professions lost their soul, spirit, and heart? One thing is sure: they typically don't have much mojo. In other words, they too often lack that unexplainable creative life force that is the root of all transformative performance. Even worse, they may have inadvertently contributed to more iatrogenesis—expanding the categories of diagnosis, perpetuating self-fulfilling prophecies concerning mental illness through media advertising, and exacerbating the patterns that maintain symptomatic role performance. Therapists too easily become disoriented and lost, forgetting that no matter what professional orientation or theoretical school is followed it won't do much good unless a therapist has a heart of healing wisdom.

In 2003, Brad was invited to speak to a packed auditorium of counselors at the annual meeting of the American Counseling Association held in Anaheim, California. Joined by Dr. William Glasser, Professor Jeffrey Kottler, and Professor Jon Carlson, he called for the mental health professions to move toward healing ways. It started a buzz in counseling circles as many letters expressed appreciation that this announcement had been publicly made. It seems many counselors and therapists were also thinking it was time to reconnect with other healing traditions and to allow wisdom to have its say.

The following year the American Counseling Association introduced the biography of Bradford Keeney, written by Jeffrey Kottler and Jon Carlson, *American Shaman: An Odyssey of Global Healing Traditions*. The book on his life won a Best Spiritual Book of 2004 Award from *Spirituality and Health* magazine. It described how his experiences with diverse global healing traditions could help direct the future practice of therapy. Originally mentored by two of the founders of cybernetics—Gregory Bateson and Heinz von Foerster —Brad became an academic director of several doctoral programs where he developed innovative approaches to systemically oriented therapy. When he left the university to launch a long-term study of healing practices, he created an encyclopedia of cultural healing traditions called *Profiles of Healing.* Brad's own autobiographical account, published in 2005, was originally called *The Gods Are Crazy*, though the publisher re-titled it, *Bushman Shaman: Awakening the Spirit Through Ecstatic Dance*. Following that work, *Shaking Medicine: The Healing Power of Ecstatic Movement*, a major historical study of diverse ecstatic healing ways, was published in 2007.

In 2008, Brad was invited to give the opening keynote address to the annual conference of the American Counseling Association in Honolulu. There he enthusiastically called for the mental health profession to awaken its healing heart. Receiving a standing ovation, his keynote address was regarded as both inspiring and controversial. Following his keynote, publishers asked him to write a book on his clinical work. *The Creative Therapist: The Art of Awakening a Session* came out in 2009.

In 2010, as endowed chair and professor at the University of Louisiana, Brad inaugurated an online doctoral program concentrating on creative systemic studies where he and Hillary teach courses in the art of creative transformation, improvisation, absurd means of change, creative forms of scholarship, and diverse healing traditions. This program supported the development of Brad's next critically celebrated book, *The Bushman Way of Tracking God*, published in 2010, and winner of a national book award, the Silver Nautilus Award.

That same year, the largest financial contributor to Transcendental Meditation, the movement responsible for helping bring meditation to the West, read Brad's books about the world's oldest ancestral culture and the original way of healing. He immediately made a commitment to help make this teaching more available to everyone. This anonymous sponsor supported our creation of a practice in the French Quarter of New Orleans. There we foster transformative experiences based on the best of old and new healing ways.

The common bond found in diverse healing traditions is their emphasis on awakening the heart, bringing practitioner and client inside a favorable climate for changing all participants. After thirty-five years of working in the arenas of cybernetics (the formal study of circularity), systemic therapy, and diverse healing traditions, Brad has joined Hillary in a major project that aims to bring forth circular therapeutics, the art of awakening the heart of healing. It draws upon the enactment of ideas and practices concerning circularity, utilization, and improvisation, doing so in ways that resonate with diverse wisdom traditions. In this book, we offer expression that attempts to both embody and evoke more transformative possibilities in clinical practice.

We want to help you get your mojo (*mojo* is a metaphor for the heart of healing - your inner resources, gifts, and wisdom) in full operation for your therapeutic practice. This is what turns your therapy into re-vitalized healing. Whether your clients experience stressful challenges, relationship issues, addictions, annoying difficulties, or simply want to step up the quality of their life and maximize their full potential, you need heartfelt mojo to bring out the best you can offer.

It is time for therapists to become traditional healers for modern times - and for clients to feel free to seek them out. We take a step toward this direction when we recognize that therapy is less a science and more an art of the heart. We are only comfortable saying that it is both an art and a science if we can also agree that the performance arts concerned with telling a joke, a magical story, or an absurd theatrical play are also science. In that case, we look forward to teaching a course on the physics of comedy, the neurobiology of theater, or the astrophysics of love. Rest assured that therapy is a form of improvisational theater and belongs in the house of performing arts. (See *The Creative Therapist: The Art of Awakening a Session, Improvisational Therapy: A Practical Guide for Creative Clinical Strategies,* and *The Flying Drum: The Mojo Doctor's Guide to Creating Magic in Your Everyday.*)

Describing and prescribing the move from therapist to healer requires more slippery and poetic expression in order to handle the paradoxes and circularities that its complexity embodies. Accordingly, throughout this book we will wear several hats including that of therapist, scholar, poet, and healer. Each orientation has a different way of voicing metaphor.

As healing poets who value therapeutic scholarship, we hope to pull your mind in multiple directions so that an opening is created, pointing you toward the passage that enables your heart to accept the call to creatively heal those who ask you for help. We will be both contradictory and paradoxical, sometimes asking you to not be a therapist in order to be more therapeutic. At other times, we will present scholarly arguments that help overthrow the hegemonies that have imprisoned heartfelt healing expression. More importantly, we will turn to poetic talk and speak to your heart, asking it to be brave and step into its rightful place as the holder and dispenser of healing wisdom. To keep us inside the performance of transformative change, all the beginning expository chapters will include ongoing examples of clinical casework.

The next chapter offers a request that may seem illogical. We are going to ask you to throw away all theories, models, and understandings of therapy. Keep in mind that many traditional healing cultures require that the student or client first purge and get cleansed before the healing medicines can be administered. Similarly, we are going to ask that you empty yourself of any overly rigid ideas that organize how you think you should behave in a session. We begin by reviewing some of the historical debates that were precipitated by calls to emphasize systemic interaction – rather than interpretation - in therapy. We discuss how even those orientations that held the most promise for bringing forth transformative interaction no longer seem to offer a way out of the seduction of theoretical narration. The art of healing requires less theoretical stasis and more changes of performed action.

We will then start introducing the wisdom ways. In Chapters 3 and 4 we shall depict the therapist's move toward healing as a leap into embodied circularity. Retracing some of the theories of circular causality that contributed to earlier so-called systemic approaches, we take a journey into the core principles of cybernetic epistemology. This latter term simply translates to circular knowing. Here knowing is created by circular patterns that link and circulate knower with known. Circularity underlies all human experience and wisdom. Its unraveling – whether in a marriage, family, clinical session, social organization, or ecosystem – pulls apart the relations that are maintained inside its circle. Circular therapeutics refers to the ways our participation in the circularity that organizes knowing and being can transform our lives, serving and healing the relational circles that hold us. At its highest realization, circular therapeutics refers to experiencing the circle of life honored by all wisdom traditions and practitioners of the healing arts.

We emphasize how both therapy and healing come alive as they are improvisationally organized by the fullest utilization of the here and now, the ongoing creation of an enriched reality that draws upon the unique offerings of what each situation presents. This performance is circular therapeutics. In the service of being cybernetic in our relationship to cybernetics, we conclude Chapter 4 with a call to go past the descriptions (and inherent limitations) of circular theory in order to bring us more fully inside the circularity it prescribes.

We then examine the ways other wisdom holders have experimented with the expression of circular embodiment in both written and performed conversational exchange. We call this "circular poetics," a way of pointing to the dedicated enactment of utilization and transformative improvisation. Specifically, the metalogues of Gregory Bateson (1972) and the Zen *koan* records of *The Gateless Gate* (Yamada, 2004) are examined in Chapter 5 as lessons in the art of embodying the paradox, absurdity, and creative complexity that accompany the expression of circular wisdom. We propose that therapy offer no less than this kind of expression - empty of reified interpretations while full of the creative presence of change. The pedagogical form of circular poetics can help teach therapists how to be more moved by the circularities of improvised interaction that can transform both client and therapist.

Chapter 6 moves us closer to the core of circular therapeutics. We explore the ways in which healing is often best kick-started through the heartfelt feeling and expression of deep emotion. Here we are not talking about the trivial sharing of personal feelings with our clients. We are pointing instead to an old teaching: the heart, which is a metaphor for the strong feeling of the biggest kind of love for and connection with others, must be awakened and expressed in order for healing to occur. Many spiritual traditions, from the Bushman healers of the Kalahari to the sanctified musicians of the old-time African-American church, teach us that the road to the heart is traveled on the waves of rhythm and song. Therapy suffers from a lack of meaningful relationship to the ineffable in human transformation, and it is evidenced by the predominant absence of authentic spirited expression in therapeutic practice. If we could sing you this chapter, we would, saying that it is not a routinized therapeutic skill but a spontaneous, heartfelt healing performance that brings forth therapeutic change.

We then introduce the voice of a traditional healer in Chapter 7 that invites therapists to go to the healing crossroads where the guiding light for circular therapeutics is found. When you are moved by the highest orders of circularity, transformative change naturally springs forth, fully guided by the deep wisdom of unconscious mind and the inspiration of inexplicable mystery.

Following these musings and poetic renderings, we provide further case examples of our work. Each case brings a teaching about circular therapeutics, the art of entering and being guided by the circularities of a healing heart. We find that the best teaching is located in the clinical work itself, and our main lessons consist of the cases that embody what is being taught.

We then step into metalogue and koanic written form to explore and generate further questions regarding the implications of moving therapy to the healing arts. We encourage the mental health professions to start emphasizing ongoing invention and creation rather than reproduction and archival replication. Otherwise, practice and knowing both stagnate and are reduced to a shallow rhetoric that carries only an echo of whatever truths were once held.

Finally, we extend an invitation to therapists to start their own journey toward embracing a healer's heart. Each therapist has an inner creative genie that is waiting to spring forth. As you move through the following pages, know that we are talking to this part of you. Inside your heart is a light that can be a beacon for others. Open the door and allow it to pour forth its boundless gifts and treasures.

There is nothing to learn; there is only one door to open. This is our only teaching. We will express it in many different ways, but each discourse is merely a knocking on the door that calls for your entry. As you turn each page, imagine that the door to healing is being opened a bit more. As it swings open, so too will your heart. This is all you need to know. The rest is mere detail.

INTERLUDE

Years ago there was a therapist who read every relevant book on how to help others. He also attended every clinical workshop offered. He was an expert on all mental health orientations from psychoanalysis to hypnosis, primal scream, family therapy, feminist therapy, and NLP. One day a most unusual client scheduled an appointment with this therapist. To his surprise, she began her first session by asking him to make up a story about his life, making sure that his fantasy emphasized how he invented a radically new therapy based on their first meeting. She meant what she said and this caught the therapist off guard. Without questioning whether he could do it, he started his tale.

"Once upon a time, I knew all the things that could be said to a client. Then a young woman came to me and asked me to make up a story about myself. I told her that I had met over a thousand clients who sat in the same chair she sat in, but that I had never heard that special request before. That's when I decided to stand up and shake her hand, saying, 'Thank you for helping me take a stand.'"

Immediately she replied, "Isn't it better to stand for action rather than sit with understanding?"

At that moment, the therapist was set free by a question that lifted his practice.

2. DELETING NARRATIVE: Purging the Internal and External Chatter

Imagine a therapist going to a Zen roshi wanting to understand more about the truth of therapy. When the therapist asks this question, the roshi answers, "Do you hear the sound of that running brook?" "Yes, I hear it," answers the therapist. "That is the entrance to the truth," the roshi replies.

Do you hear the sound of the stream of life, the flow experience that is moving us along? Inside that stream is found not only the life of a session, but all important situational truths arise in its ongoing flux. What we are looking for is how to be more presently engaged inside this stream, where the stream itself can be utilized. Working with the flow of life is more advantageous than opposing it. The latter commences when we construe a dissociated narrative that disembodies us, and through a kind of out-of-body experience we fantasize ourselves on the bank of the stream. There we assume a narrator's position, looking at life and therapy through a theoretical account, story, map, or reflection as the stream is assumed to be observed from afar. In this fragmented state of affairs, we serve the reflecting mirage, suggesting that the territory is distant and unknowable. In this delusion, we erroneously assume that we have to settle for living in a map, never again able to return to the stream. This attachment to story and interpretation is the root of suffering, or so advise many of the longstanding wisdom traditions. Our invitation to purge narrative is an invitation to become less dissociated inside a delusional mirage, and jump back into the embodied stream, waking up to remember that you never left it all along.

Here we prepare you to take a stand against therapy theories that so often become obstacles to therapeutic presence. We essentially invite you to be free and tap into your own creative processes, moving from the routines of therapy to a heartfelt embodiment of healing—the art of performing circular therapeutics. Please recognize that you are being offered release from the stranglehold of any theoretical explanation (including those surrounding "healing") that seduces both therapists and clients into thinking either human suffering or transformation can be adequately understood, or that there must first be diagnostic understanding before acting to help others. We are also freeing you from the imprisonment of any and all models of therapy. Though they tickle our imaginations when they are first conceived, they quickly turn into shackles that retard creative expression, fostering worn-out, clichéd habits of action.

In other words, we invite you to let go of all attachment to what you think you know or need to know, including any fixated search for problems, solutions, patterns of interaction, internalizations, externalizations, narratives, or any meaning behind anything you encounter in a clinical session. We do this as a skillful means for interrupting all prevailing therapeutic orientations that suggest suffering can be transformed through uncovering more understanding, altering stories, or co-constructing preferred interpretations about a client's experience. Purge yourself of the inner and outer clinical chatter that distracts you from hearing the heartbeat of healing.

Debates in therapy—especially family and brief therapies—are primarily organized around the choice between approaching clients as an observing narrator versus being a more spontaneously involved participant guided by the here-and-now movement of our interactions with one another. In other words, do you get caught deliberating over reflections, hypotheses, interpretations, or narratives or are you more inclined to act first in order to see what happens to kick-start the improvisational flow of interaction? Are you caught in an out-of-body narration on the bank of the stream, or are you in the stream itself?

At the time Keeney (1983) wrote *Aesthetics of Change*, the leading metaphors "cybernetics," "ecosystemic" and "systemic" had come to designate the paradigmatic shift in family therapy from the psychodynamic emphasis on analysis and interpretation to an emphasis on systemic interaction. Here the action of every participant in an interactional system was seen as interwoven with the action of all participants. The therapeutic focus was on being inside the interactional stream. Since every action was a cause of every other action, the interpretive search for a problem's origin was rendered irrelevant. Changing any action of any participant could result in change throughout the whole system. Here a family member's attempted solutions were also interactional problems, while problems could sometimes be regarded as interactional solutions. Treating a whole family, including praising a symptom bearer while expressing concern about the presumed wellness and success of non-symptom bearers, made therapeutic sense when circular interactivity was emphasized.

Cybernetics provides a precise means of specifying the circular interactions that hold communicative performance. The word itself comes from a Greek word meaning "the art of steering." In its simplest definition, it is about having a goal and the kind of action needed to achieve that goal. In therapy, the goal is to help a client move from impoverished to enriched experience. To reach this goal, you have to continuously check how close you are getting to it. You must constantly circulate the difference between where you are and where you want to be in order to get there. Called feedback, this constant monitoring of change keeps on re-specifying how to act, doing so from moment to moment. Act to reach your goal, notice the difference that results, and utilize that difference to act differently (that is, change your behavior) in order to try reaching your goal again.

Cybernetics emphasizes the circular process of constantly changing one's action in order to serve change. It also frees us from the idea that suffering is caused by one isolated element, whether it is identified as a pathogenic cortex, inadequate learned response, inappropriate social coalition, or oppressive cultural narrative. Cybernetics emphasizes how you handle your choice of action, rather than prescribes any particular action or routine. It does so to help therapy move toward its course of helping change the way clients relate to suffering. Non-cybernetic models offer fixed plot lines rather than circularities of ongoing change. A typical therapy model begins by explaining what is wrong and then prescribes the sequential steps to correct it. Cybernetics, with its appreciation that all things are circularly organized, asks you to act independent of a script. Act in order to find out how to act next, doing so inside the stream of interactivity, without succumbing to the temptation to exit toward sideline narration.

Note that when we regard a cybernetic circularity as separate from our observing, we are participating in first-order cybernetics. But when the cybernetician is brought inside the circularity, the re-circulation of the observer into the observed marks second-order cybernetics. First-order fulfills sideline narration, commenting on what it observes; whereas second-order is found in the stream of action, more organized by non-narrated interactivity. Suffice it to say that we are not indicating anything more with this distinction than what the Zen roshi attempts to communicate when pointing to a stream when a therapist asks any question.

Whatever groundbreaking interactional difference so-called systemic therapies once offered was short-lived. For a brief historical moment, there was a clearly distinguished break from therapeutic habits of incessant interpretation and instead a focus on systemic circularity, with an invitation to be more change oriented, doing so inside the flow of interaction. Therapists primarily acted in order to help change a system while limiting their diagnosis to observing how the system responded to their efforts to change them. Subsequent therapeutic action utilized outcomes to guide and fine-tune their next attempts to initiate change.

This way of interacting in order to facilitate change soon became challenged by a backlash of interpreters—therapy as an interactional, systemic dance faded as the notion of "systemic" regressed to another way of interpreting rather than enacting. The story of how family therapy's promise for a mental health revolution became hijacked is a detective story in itself. We will present a few details of that story in order to set a context that makes clear what was lost when the systemic emphasis on interaction was pulled out of the stream to take up residency with disembodied interpreters who narrate rather than participate.

In other words, though there has been a lot of discourse about systems, there has been little sustained embodiment of systemic practice. In particular, cybernetics was grossly misunderstood by advocates and critics alike. As professor of cybernetics, Klaus Krippendorff (2012), summarizes this history: "When therapists discovered cybernetics, many started using its vocabulary without living up to its promises." Paradoxically, the field's misunderstanding of cybernetics largely arose when it was emphasized as another description for understanding therapy rather than a prescription for organizing more circular participation in the performance of therapy.

Most therapists took the familiar psychological road, with the result that many schools of family therapy fell back into a form of individual therapy where the family either served as an interpretive backdrop for a client's (and therapist's) understanding, or as an audience to observe the therapist work with each member in a psychological way. The same is true today. It should be no surprise that professional ownership of family therapy is contested by clinical psychology, counseling, and marriage and family therapy. If psychiatric diagnosis, naïve positivism, narrative interpretation, and psychological explanations (including neurobiology) are accommodated by all competitors, then there is nothing distinctly systemic offered by any.

A critique of the profession is offered as a means of helping identify and liberate some of the unnecessary constraints underlying diverse schools of systemic and post-systemic therapies. Concerned that those who fail to recognize history are doomed to repeat it, we scrutinize some of the prohibitions, limiting assumptions, and arbitrary restrictions that impede the creative advance of therapeutic expression. We need to be more aware of the roots of our tradition's mishaps and misadventures to help set us free from any habits that dampen the delivery of therapeutic change that diverse voices may deliver. A more generative future for therapy benefits from going past the logjams of some of the earlier debates and highlighting what we feel is the most crucial distinction: the shift from interpretative narrativity to improvisational performance guided by interactivity. The latter brings us into the enactment of more circular, less reductive and dualistic ways of knowing found in many healing traditions.

DID THE MENTAL RESEARCH INSTITUTE LOSE ITS "MIND" TO "POWER"?

One theoretical, paradigmatic difference did arise during the early history of family therapy. This change of perspective came from the Mental Research Institute. Following Gregory Bateson (1972), an original member of the Macy meetings that gave conceptual birth to cybernetics, the researchers at the Mental Research Institute in Palo Alto, California, mostly limited themselves to cybernetic, communicational, and systems theories. Their choice of institute name was a departure from conventional family therapy rhetoric, abandoning a primary emphasis upon the sociological metaphor of "family." Bateson's influence on their choice of an alternative metaphor is obvious, as he had previously launched the call for an emphasis upon "mind" as a way of talking about the cybernetic organization of communication.

Of course there was no homeostasis surrounding any single idea within the Palo Alto ranks. Don Jackson (1957, 1965) originally described the family as a homeostatic self-regulating system, while Paul Watzlawick, John Weakland, and Richard Fisch (1974) later developed a model that highlighted the circular organization of problems and attempted solutions. Though it wasn't their primary claim, their ideas can be regarded as a simple cybernetic model of therapy that was not reliant upon either sociological or psychological frameworks. The family was only part of the interactional system if its members played a part in attempted solutions, problem definitions, or the context surrounding either.

Another orientation arose with Jay Haley's advocacy for a model of power relations, social hierarchy concerns, and coalitionary enactment. He left Palo Alto for Philadelphia where he joined Minuchin and Montalvo, developing a more sociological systems approach—Minuchin's (1974) structural family therapy and Haley's (1976a) problem solving therapy. They were essentially the same practice of power brokering, differing only in that Haley used more communicational metaphors in his theory.

Bateson (1972, 1974) despised the metaphor of power, seeing it as obscuring the patterns of interaction that do not require the extrapolation of either the internal motivations of intrapsychic processes or assumed "forces" in a social field. He proposed "mind" as an alternative to "power." It is ironic that the Mental Research Institute followed his use of "mind" in their name, but remained distinct from Bateson's emphasis upon regarding mind as an alternative to the "power" metaphor. This likely stemmed from the importance the MRI clinicians gave to a therapist orchestrating "influence" on their clients. Already in their beginning formulations of interaction, attributes of motivation were seeping into the theoretical accounts—communication became an attempt to "define," "influence," and even express "power" in relationship. Bateson was more than a scholarly pedantic wanting to be ostentatious in the way cybernetic metaphor was handled. He regarded cybernetics as a paradigmatic difference that lost its difference as soon as the old habits of discourse re-entered. This was especially the case for using the metaphor of power when connoting interaction, for it shifts the emphasis away from circularly organized patterns, while at the same time highlights an interpretation of the interaction rather than the interactivity itself.

To briefly review Bateson's (1972) position, he argued that the belief in power—whether you thought you had it or not—was a potentially toxic way of punctuating human experience. It resulted in power games on both sides of a troublesome interaction. Here the posturing of "power tactics" against an aggressor maintains unilateral action "against" the other, doing so at the cost of feeding both parties' placement inside an escalating vicious cycle of self-fulfilling verification—a debilitating game with no escape. But deleting "power" as an explanatory metaphor does not render one blind to the abuses of inequality, nor does it mean that the relational dynamics we explain through "power" do not exist. Instead it makes clearer the interactional processes that maintain them.

When a king demands that his subjects pay unfair taxes or else be thrown in a dungeon, we need not say more than this interaction embodies an inequality of social relations that helps maintain unfair law. Adding the notion of "power" contributes nothing to our understanding or ability to alter the interaction. Similarly, we are not enlightened by saying that the king has too much "one-up gusto," "leadership enzymes," "kingish gamma rays," or "big boy toxins." The latter metaphors, along with the notion of power, actually serve to mystify the king as owning some quality, essence, or social force field that makes it less possible for his subjects to do something about the situation. Limiting ourselves to discerning a "difference in equality" reminds us that it is "difference" rather than mysterious substances and forces like power or destiny that maintain the interaction. There is more room for change when we face "difference" than any elusive and invisible "power." The former can be altered by creative strategic differences that make a difference.

Highlighting "interaction" rather than "power" is not a simplistic transference of fault or "shared blame." It is an invitation to have more choice of action inside problematic situations, including those that are organized by inequality. When therapists cling to the importance of "power" in their descriptions, explanations, and tactics, they risk contributing to the way this metaphor coaxes a client into either feeling more helpless and without choice, or limited to the choice of engaging in eye-for-an-eye power games. Power overshadows the interactional complexity involved in human relational contexts. Those seen as "having no power" are able to make choices inside the contexts of their lives that can make a difference, even when those choices are severely limited. This has led to the resiliency and survival of people and cultures across generations under colonialism, apartheid, and other forms of violence. There is nothing liberating or therapeutic about a theory that allows a metaphor like power to reduce, mystify, or make invisible the possibilities for creative choice inside difficult situations.

Whereas Gandhi proposed that all violence was evil and advocated non-cooperation and peaceful resistance, Bateson (1972) argued all notions of power—when applied to human relations—were harmfully erroneous. He advocated nonparticipation and noncooperation in the making of descriptions, explanations, or premises that were derivative of the metaphor of power. Family therapy, narrative therapy, and postmodern therapy never heard or responded to Bateson's call. It was as radical a challenge as the proponents of nonviolence must have seemed to social movements wanting to fight their oppressors with equivalent conceptual and physical tools.

Bateson was discouraged by how he saw the metaphor of power organizing theories and practices of family therapy—especially when they also bantered about the metaphors of communication, systems, mind, and cybernetics—the very ideas that he saw as an alternative to thinking in terms of power. This disappointing confoundment contributed to his leaving the entire field and dissociating himself from its proponents. Haley, in particular, made light of Bateson's argument and tried to hide it from the field as being irrelevant (Bateson, Weakland, & Haley, 1976). When Haley (1961/1976b) published his account of the Bateson research team, Bateson (as cited in Harries-Jones, 1995) sent a letter to him saying:

> For me it brings back all the bitterness and agony of being unable to get my point across to you. I guess you thought that every move I made was a 'power' play. I assumed, of course, that a year or two of working in our project would be sufficient to convince you that 'power' is a cultural myth based upon an anti-cybernetic position . . . (p. 272)

The Bateson-Haley conflict was a turning point in the field's history. Though covered up as if it were a family secret, this heated controversy and professional divorce meant that one of the most important theorists responsible for providing family therapy with its original cybernetic and systemic ideas dissociated from his formerly close colleagues, believing they had misappropriated the shift suggested by "mental research."

Meanwhile, conflict between Watzlawick and Bateson led to an equally painful separation. Bateson had been writing his ideas for a book when *Pragmatics of Human Communication* (Watzlawick, Beavin, & Jackson, 1967) was published. The latter was largely an assemblage of ideas and illustrations

Bateson wished to present in his own work. Bateson felt they had not been correctly presented by Watzlawick and, worse, believed that his work had been stolen (Harries-Jones, 1995, p. 27). More specifically, in 1961, Bateson planned a landmark contribution that would provide a communicative exploration of schizophrenia, metaphor, humor, and paradox. The manuscript was ready in 1965, "but was pre-empted by members and associates of his own research team" (Harries-Jones, 1995, p. 27). Norton, the publisher with whom Bateson had a book contract, had made a deal with these authors behind Bateson's back. Feeling discouraged over seeing his own theoretical work stolen and misrepresented by someone else, Bateson never finished the book he intended. Years later Haley reported that Pragmatics "took the basic ideas of the Bateson project and did not give proper credit for them" and "reported Bateson as saying that the book stole 30 of his ideas" (Harries-Jones, 1995, p. 27). Bateson (as cited in Harries-Jones, 1995) wrote Watzlawick an angry letter saying among other things that, "I used to wonder how the Kahunas [Hawaiian priests] feel when they see the carvings of their gods in the shop window of a travel bureau. Now I know. . . And the loot is sometimes correctly labeled as provenance. And the native has no comeback" (p. 28). And so it came to be that Bateson's desired aesthetic holding of these ideas was usurped and delivered to the profession inside Watzlawick, Beavin, and Jackson's (1967) pragmatic reframe.

Keeney (1982, 1983) brought up the historic controversy over the metaphor of power and the reframing of Bateson's aesthetic ideas as pragmatic in the early 1980s and was predictably attacked by the guardians of MRI, including Watzlawick in a feature issue of *Family Process* (volume 29, issue 4) that highlighted this critique. More than a decade later at an Ericksonian conference in Orlando where Watzlawick, Keeney, and Sophie Freud sat on a panel together, Keeney told Watzlawick that Bateson, though previously hurt, had later endorsed his book on change and problem solving in the *Whole Earth Catalogue*. After all those years of estrangement from his mentor, Watzlawick expressed gratitude upon hearing this affirmation, lamenting how he never understood why Bateson had felt betrayed by him because he had, after all, dedicated the book to him.

Family therapy has always been an extraordinarily dysfunctional family. Perhaps this is always true for human groups, but it is particularly so for the cast of characters that made up our history. The early marriage of the field to the metaphor of power bred a discipline that valued the art of one-upmanship, and this arguably played itself out not only in its therapies but also in its professional discourse. Social interaction was too often reduced to power tactics, and the cybernetic promise of an alternative interactional metaphor of circular mind was never brought into the mainstream. Worse, therapists were hindered from going past the constraints of narrative interpretation and traversing the circular pathways that lead to the heart of healing transformation.

THE UNDOING OF CIRCULARITY IN SYSTEMIC FAMILY THERAPY: THE HOFFMAN BLUNDER

It seems the family therapy field (as well as narrative and postmodern therapies) has not always had a sufficient grasp of the ideas and theories that it mentions in its writings and teachings. An intellectual investigation awaits a scholar who can detail how cybernetics and systems theories have been misunderstood by both its proponents and critics. It would include showing how proponents of simple cybernetics clung to an interpretation of interaction rather than submitting to improvisational interactivity. Consider Haley's (1976b) claim that a social system has a "need for power"—this psychological interpretation of social organization (making the latter an upsized individual) shows how far astray his thinking went from the emphasis on interactional pattern prescribed by cybernetics. In addition, the postmodern advocates of higher order cybernetics never embodied its circularity, but favored interpretive discourse that underscored endless commentary, reflection, conversation, and description of observations and observations of observations. The major proponents of collaborative conversation and inclusion paradoxically became more removed from the interactive domain. The more they talked about second-order cybernetics, dialogue, and co-construction, the less they enacted it.

During the late 70's and early 80's, a controversy took place in the field of family therapy that resulted in a political frenzy that changed the course of the profession. It began when Brad spent a week in 1976 with Gregory Bateson in Ben Lomond, California, interviewing him about his work in psychotherapy. There Bateson shared his personal correspondence with Haley, Watzlawick and others who had been involved with him during the time he was working in Palo Alto. The controversies that surrounded their relationships and work led Bateson to feeling angry, sad, and even betrayed. Bateson lamented that he largely left the mental health professions due to his being hurt by his associates. The situation was compounded because the same people he broke relations with cited him as their intellectual mentor and used his academic reputation to help legitimize their work. Even today, Gregory Bateson is often seen as associated with the work of the Mental Research Institute and most communication-oriented approaches to therapy. Brad, being a graduate student in his twenties, witnessed Bateson's confession of pain as he heard that those who robbed and distorted his thinking also claimed that his ideas were the foundation of their way of working. Bateson went as far to say to Brad that, "The only sane response would have been to have gone screaming and running naked down the street."

Keeney publicly discussed the theoretical differences between Bateson and the MRI associates when he was Director of Research at the Ackerman Institute of Family Therapy. In a yearlong course on clinical epistemology, one of the attendees was his colleague, Lynn Hoffman, who was also at Ackerman. When Lynn Hoffman heard about this previously unreported dispute, she immediately recognized its importance. Brad did not share all the details concerning the matters of plagiarism Bateson had with Watzlawick. That report was later brought to the public by Harries-Jones (1995) and substantiated by Bateson's archival letters.

During Brad's years at the Ackerman Institute, he and Lynn Hoffman had many conversations about the falling-out between Bateson and the therapists from MRI, especially about Bateson's concern for the metaphor of power. She credits Brad as having brought her attention to this dispute and its historical importance (Hoffman, 1993b), but her rendition and understanding of the controversy became reshaped in a way that has been overlooked. She does not free herself from the use of power as Bateson proposed, but instead throws away the very interactional circularity that is the heart of Bateson's cybernetics. The result is that she removes herself from systemic thinking and subsequently pronounces that therapists need to embrace interpretation rather than circular interactivity as their primary orientation. Furthermore, she makes this shift with the claim that she is following Bateson and other so-called second-order cyberneticians. Like Bateson's previous colleagues, she uses his name to legitimize the very ideas he was against. In no way is Bateson's epistemology not cybernetic—he called it cybernetic epistemology. Nor is second-order cybernetics not cybernetic. The latter is doubly cybernetic! Hoffman's catapult out of Batesonian epistemology, while claiming to be an ambassador for it, unfortunately became the map that charted the future course of family therapy, especially with the development of the soon to follow narrative and postmodern models, both of which misappropriated Bateson and second-order cybernetics in the same way enacted by Hoffman.

How did family therapy become a second-order power narrative (another round of emphasizing the importance of power as metaphor and explanation) rather than the fulfillment and embodiment of second-order cybernetics? It most likely had something to do with politics. Brad always regarded Hoffman's (1985/1993a, 1993b) use of Bateson's differentiation from MRI to be inspired by something personal, as if she had an ax to grind. Her overly simplistic description of the reified "mechanistic-oriented therapist" as less than human, being a mere technological agent of control with little sensitivity to diversity and relational dynamics, sounds more like a rant than an indication of how the therapists she criticizes may have themselves misunderstood and possibly misapplied cybernetic thinking. Without hypothesizing the reasons for why Hoffman went from one extreme to another—from being an enthusiastic cheerleader for the ideas and therapists she later caustically chastises—her criticism has the unfortunate consequence of creating more muddle than clarity.

What matters is that a major difference re-entered the field when Brad brought back Bateson's critique of power-oriented ways of interpreting human interaction. As MRI had misappropriated Bateson's epistemology, Hoffman (1985/1993a, 1993b) did the same, but this time went further. While MRI at least retained the importance of circular interactivity, Hoffman threw the baby out with the bathwater. In so doing it appeared that she was trying to discard the contributions of the early pioneers who had made the important emphasis of interaction over narrative, or what we call the primacy of performed circularity over interpretation.

This moment in family therapy history did not go unnoticed by astute observers of the field. Glenn Collins, a reporter from the *New York Times*, sensed that the field was on the edge of making history, while at the same time was confused about the differences it was delivering. He asked Brad to be the key informant for a book about the profession he planned to write, since Brad was in the middle of many of the important controversies and conversations. Being more of a theorist at the time, he was not allegiant to any particular model. This position gave Brad access to many of the pioneer therapists who shared their outlooks with him. He had a unique insider's view of the conversations that were shaping the field. Over several years, Glenn followed Brad to numerous conferences and held personal interviews that were tape-recorded. Due to the illness of Glenn's father and Brad's leaving New York City for an academic position in Texas, they abandoned the project. Recently, however, this archival material has been released, serving as the data for a historical study conducted by Brooke Keels (in press).

It is worth noting that Hoffman was not principally regarded as a clinician during this period, but as a reporter, historian, and commentator on other people's work. She has never been as well known for a particular therapy session as she is for her narratives about therapy in general. As Brad recalls, she frequently shied away from performing cases in public view, and when she began doing that she did so with the caveat that she was not a charismatic character who could influence change. What took place in her writing that came years later, however, was that she claimed to evolve the understanding that "good therapy" was the kind of work that looked more like a conversation where the therapist did not try to bring forth change.

Another of Brad's colleagues and close friends, Harry Goolishian, was also a friend of Hoffman. He too was fond of minimizing his presence in a session, typically doing so with a wonderful sense of humor. He often joked that a "good session" was a boring session. Brad used to tease Harry saying, "Just because your sessions are boring, doesn't mean they are good." Goolishian, like Hoffman, later created a model of therapy that minimized the importance of trying to create change, instead proposing being a minimal participant in a conversation. As an observer of all these therapists, Brad began wondering whether less skilled (or less active, or less performative) clinicians favored models that advance doing less. It validated the way they performed. There is nothing wrong with that until it becomes a moral outcry against those whose skills or approach result in more alive sessions and more apparent change.

It isn't surprising that Brian Stagoll (2000) implied that the popularity of narrative therapy took place because it enabled therapists to no longer have to go through the ordeal and intense learning required to be an interactive participant in helping others change. He went further to ponder, "I sometimes wonder if it has not been a massive retreat from interaction that has led us into getting lost" (Stagoll, 2000, p. 5). In the renaissance of interpretation privileged over interactivity, a therapist could do nothing while having a theory that reframes lack of skill or the paucity of significant action as the indication of mastery. In the case of family therapy, various schools of practice were launched by the opening manipulative maneuver of lambasting cybernetics, while claiming to authorize their new alternatives as examples of second-order cybernetics (Hoffman, 1985/1993a, 1993b). They offered a disconnect from cybernetics and circularity, and offered instead, an exaltation of interpretation.

The denigration of cybernetics, articulated by Hoffman (1985/1993a, 1993b, 2002) and then continued by others, including Anderson (1997), was a kind of shape-shifting sophistry that masked what was actually going on: throwing away interactivity (particularly circular interactivity) in order to return to narrative interpreting. As therapists were struggling to understand what a systemic, interactional, and cybernetic approach to therapy entailed, Hoffman (1993b) offered the ostensible definition of "second order" as the practice of a "removed" observer self-reflecting about their interpretations. In her own words:

> This term [second order] comes from mathematics and merely means taking a position that is a step removed from the operation itself so that you can perceive the operation reflexively. These views are really views about views... allow[ing] you to see that a particular interpretation is only one among many possible versions. (Hoffman, 1993b, p. 91)

Hoffman (1993b) goes on to argue that this is the second-order "lens" that was later applied to cybernetics. While second-order cybernetics agrees that an observer is capable of making many possible observations, its basic point is to emphasize the circularity between observer and the observed (Keeney, 1983). The concept of second order is not a simple invitation to shift one's attention to a bird's-eye view that now observes both therapist and client (Hoffman, 1985/1993a), but rather how neither therapist nor client can ever take a "step removed" (Hoffman, 1993b, p. 91) position from his or her circle of interaction. Here we emphasize neither staring at the observed nor the observer—it is not a change in a viewing stance as Hoffman argues. Second-order cybernetics doubles the notion of circularity, enabling cybernetics to emphasize the constant re-entries of the indicating cybernetician into the circularities that are of interest.

Hoffman (1985/1993a, 1993b) further debased cybernetics by her misconstrued articulations of its basic terms, such as "control," which in her discourse becomes defined as a desire for unilateral control over or manipulation of others, rather than a way of indicating a system's organizational stability. Would we criticize a dancer whose "control" of physical movement enables grace to be expressed? Under Hoffman's observing eye, Martha Graham could be belittled for her desire for unilateral control or manipulation of the movement of a dancer, not seeing that freedom of expression includes skilled control of motion. Her criticism of the early systemic models of family therapy would be comedic if it weren't for the fact that other therapists took it seriously, as she demonized interactively organized therapists as controlling masterminds who regard families as "trivial machines" (Hoffman, 1993b, p. 92) who can be manipulated (Hoffman, 1985/1993a, pp. 10-32 , Hoffman, 1993b, p. 36).

Hoffman (1993) missed the more important point that all models of therapy, by virtue of being a model, treat people as trivially organized. This is as true for postmodern and narrative models as it is for the models they critique. What is lost in Hoffman's falling out of cybernetic circularity is the originating experience that inspired the field of family therapy. Inspired by the work of Harry Goolishian and Harlene Anderson (see Hoffman, 1993b, p. 83), she brought us back to the archaic notion that classical hermeneutics should triumph over postmodern participation in the real-time choreography of live interaction.

Hoffman (1993b) and the family therapists who relied on her interpretations threw away both circularity and interaction, and pronounced that second-order cybernetics was an invitation to interpretive relativism and self-reflection. Her leap is nothing more than moving from "observing the observed" to "observing the observer," failing to realize that the latter is nothing more than a first order shift that makes the observer the observed. Rather than underscoring that "observing observing" points to a recursive interaction, Hoffman's sleight of hand unwinds the double circularity of second-order circularity and returns us back to navel gazing and endless babbling about biases and self-reflections, all done without mention of the relevance of an ongoing circular flow of interactive process. Stuck in self-reflexive gazing, the reflections of mirroring therapists brought them closer to psychoanalysts and Rogerian counselors, and further away from the interactional dynamics that almost started a new revolution for the mental health professions. In a single stroke, Hoffman and her lineage of observers and reflectors sleight and make disappear the most important contribution of family therapy and cybernetics—circular interactivity. This mishap, call it the Hoffman blunder, resulted in the unwinding of circularity in systemic family therapy.

Second-order cybernetics' contribution is in how it helps keep a person inside the circularities that are indicated/constituted/expressed in an ongoing interaction. As Gordon Pask (1996), one of the pioneers of cybernetics indicated, second-order cybernetics emphasizes participant observers that interact. In summary, first order cybernetics is the first indication of circularity, first accomplished at the cost of amnesia, that is, forgetting, that we are indicating the circularity. Second-order cybernetics is a wake up call that brings back the remembrance that we are being circulated by circularity as we indicate it.

In therapy, this is a reminder that the observation of pathology, problems, solutions, resources, patterns of interaction, narratives, and meanings are inseparable from the actions of the therapist. Second-order therapy is not a stampede toward interpretation, non-action, and witnessed stories. It is the therapy of therapy. Whereas the first order circularity of family therapy was defined as a therapist utilizing the outcomes of her efforts to change a client, second-order circularity utilizes the results of these interactions to change the therapist's way of participating. When therapy is applied to itself, it changes. Therapy models unfortunately do not encourage outcome based interaction with themselves, that is, they do not double back to include themselves as the subject of their operations. Instead they act as if the model is outside the therapist, client, and session. The very idea of a therapy model, whether called strategic or narrative, is a first-order notion. It exists to maintain itself, doing so by maintaining the distance of observing.

Relying on Hoffman's (1993b, 2002) voice as historian, the advocates of interpretation disguised as proponents of systemic therapy became a chorus that rivaled any nonsense Lewis Carroll ever conceived. Here "systemic" loses its interactional emphasis and higher order cybernetics contains no cybernetics at all. Joining the tea party, White and Epston (1990) essentially announced that Bateson didn't actually offer a systemic view, but rather an "interpretive method" (p. 2) in which knowing is the process of making sense of events through the construction of maps and narratives. This reductionism and reversal of Bateson's position seems to imply that any liberty can be taken when we interpret. Their claim that "since we cannot know objective reality, all knowing requires an act of interpretation" (p. 2), perhaps has been over applied to their reading of Bateson, as if they are saying, "since we cannot know Bateson, all knowing about his ideas allows us to take any liberty we want in interpreting him." Bateson insisted on the importance of behavioral description to keep our abstractions from getting too far removed from experience, the relational specification (in interactional terms) of context, the embodiment of a cybernetic organization of knowing, and the emphasis on the difference between a map and territory. His work becomes completely scrambled in White and Epston's highly questionable "translation" that insists on minimizing an acknowledgment of the present action scene, equating the premises of mapping as a specification of context, and the advocacy of mapped interpretation rather than the circulated difference that makes a difference across the interface between map and territory. White et al. severely dilute, distort, and vulgarize Bateson's (1972) nuanced handling of logical typing, context and communication, and the epistemological process of drawing distinctions, doing so to advance their non-systemic, non-cybernetic emphasis on naïve narrative meaning making.

It is not uncommon for therapists to misrepresent Bateson's ideas while claiming to base their work upon him. In one historical study of the influence of Gregory Bateson on family therapy, Thomas, Waits, and Hartfield (2007) make clear that Bateson has become more vestige than legacy. They found that while family therapy authors often make a reference to Bateson, it seems directed to adding authority to their own credibility since there is rarely any connection to his ideas or way of thinking. Pakman (2004, p. 423) even claimed that the field should honor Bateson's "spirit" and not his "letter." Whatever that means, it likely is exemplified by how Pakman references Bateson and other cyberneticians while advocating a therapy that serves interpretation rather than interactive performance. Finally, Thomas et al. point out that a Family Process issue published in 2004 as a dedication to Bateson's work finds only two articles even referencing Bateson, with neither having any relation to his epistemological orientation.

Worshipping the Almighty Throne of Interpretive Discourse

What happened to the field of family therapy, with few exceptions, is that cybernetics and systemic metaphors were usurped and translated as another form of interpretation, and the epistemological leap into cybernetic recursivity was never made. In this parade of anti-cybernetic confusion and logical mistyping, therapists and clients are domesticated once again by the tyranny of the narrator who now claims to offer a more liberating, postmodern, and collaborative form of interpretation. Interpretive relativity is still interpretation after all, and it makes king or queen of the narrator sitting outside and passing judgment on the circles of interaction where cyberneticians, interactional therapists, and traditional healers serve the processes of transformation by being inside them, rather than lording over them as a meta-reflecting, moralistic editor.

Heinz von Foerster's (1984) postmodern cybernetic invitations to "act in order to know" and to "act so as to increase the number of choices" were sidelined as post-systemic (though called postmodern) therapies called for no action in therapy (Anderson, 1997). Responsibility for action that promoted change was minimized in favor of less action and knowing—don't act in order to not know. Enactment, action, interaction, and intervention became taboo words. The field returned to where therapy had begun—worshipping the almighty throne of interpretive discourse. It was as if interactional and earlier systemic therapies never existed. Therapy recycled to the beginning—the production of theory, story, commentary, reflection, hypothesis, and narrative.

The movement from Freudian explanation to postmodern and postcolonial reflection required a middle transition, and it was supplied by the contribution of the Milan approach to systemic family therapy. The Milan psychoanalytically trained team reinterpreted the family's story in a way that provided a new meaning of family dynamics, hoping it would paradoxically initiate a change. Their work was distanced from the more interactionally organized improvisational flow of a therapist less organized by any desire to reach the climax of a grand interpretation.

It was no accident that the propagandist for interpreting therapies, Lynn Hoffman (1985/1993a, 2002), insinuated that both the Milan work and later postmodern approaches were more "systemic" and more "higher order cybernetic" than their predecessors. She framed their emergence as representative of an ongoing evolution of therapy. Her polemics set the stage for implicitly declaring, whether she meant to or not, that interpretation had conquered interactivity and that the "best theory" (and the idea that there is a "best meta-narrative") ruled once again. A more systemically oriented historian might have depicted the field's chronological performances as a devolution of systemic and cybernetic embodiment.

Therapists - no matter how long they have been practicing - are easily distracted by the idea that correct understanding by therapist and/or client will lead to change. Whether cast as reflection, hypothesis, dialogue, or narrative, it is assumed that therapy is best delivered through the way interpretive commentary is given space and handled. Call it re-authoring of a story, a dialogical dance, a polyphonic carnival of multi-storied discourse, or a conversational realm of handling difference, it comes down to mediating change through the management of construed, reconstrued, deconstrued, and misconstrued understanding.

In this semantically driven universe, Freud, Bateson, and Foucault, among others, are reduced to being interpretive choices. Here the contested ground of therapy is situated in a competition for the dominant way of understanding, again including those who claim conversational relativity while advancing a right way to handle the different understandings. This framing of the profession's context makes therapists blind to an alternative choice that goes beyond the arena of diverse interpretations.

NARRATIVITY AND INTERACTIVITY:
THE DIFFERENCE THAT MAKES A DIFFERENCE

The more critical distinction is between narrativity and interactivity. The latter is not easy to grasp for a culture whose *modus operandi* stems from "know in order to know how to act." Here understanding precedes action and right understanding brings correct action. The paradigmatic flip brought by what we call embodied cybernetics (once called "second-order cybernetics" or the "cybernetics of cybernetics") was precisely the opposite. Acting in order to know how to act in the next moment is the nature of improvisational conduct. It is born of the moment and is self-generating. We propose that cybernetics and improvisation are two kindred metaphors for this kind of interactivity.

The "interactional view" of Watzlawick, Weakland, and Fisch of the

Mental Research Institute in Palo Alto should have not said "view" for it, too, tempts us to view rather than do. It would have been clearer and less a semantic trap if they had advocated "interactional performance," "interactional participation," or "interactional pragmatics."

The leading designers of video games center their intellectual arguments on whether games should be built from a narrative or interactive basis. Their discussions refer to the "narrativity versus interactivity" debate. The same distinction has always been inherent in the field of therapy, but it has not been an overt part of the conversations, debates, and politics. Keeney and Ross (1985) proposed that this distinction underlies all debates regarding therapy and called it the difference between semantics (meaning) and politics ("politics" referring to the "who-is-doing-what-to-whom-when-where-and-how," i.e., interactivity). A therapist either primarily serves interpretations or improvisationally inspired interaction. Though both are always present, the primacy of meaning and narrative too easily masks the interactivity that generates storytelling and meaning making. The holding of meaning inside interactivity helps prevent the client and therapist from disembodying themselves and their stories from the ongoing interaction.

Stated differently, the embodiment of interactivity includes interpretations, but they are invented for each unique situation. While interpreting and storying always remain in a field of interactive performance, its exaltation to being the focus of therapy fails because it cannot escape promoting (on some level) a preferred discourse—it helps others "discover" the correct, better, freer story that gives improved meaning to their life. Here liberation consciousness is operationalized as a therapist's imposition of metaphors that reduce clients' experience to the therapist's definition of social oppression (e.g., dynamics related to gender, culture, race, etc.), and the clichéd, redundant asking of permission and habituated questions are seen as respect—all done with no self-reflexive awareness that all scripted talk has the smell of inauthentic presence as a therapist obediently follows rule-governed conduct. In spite of any well-meaning intention, these formulaic therapies too easily enact the imposition of ideology that narrative and postmodern approaches claim to avoid. We must avoid colonizing anyone with any idea or therapy model—even anti-colonial ones—no matter how right it might seem to us. Conducting therapy from a platform of any liberation theory easily risks undoing the contribution to liberation it seeks (see Keeney & Keeney's essay, "Externalization in Narrative Therapy: Addressing a Modernist Re-Emergence of Exorcism," 2012a). We best serve the highest ideals by sometimes not pushing them onto others. This is wisdom know-how rather than naïve knowing-it-all.

When the map becomes the territory, as it does for all models—we end up with paradoxical reversals where the intended outcome of a model creates its opposite. Hence, Watzlawick, Weakland, and Fisch present an interactional view that becomes another interpretive model of interactional understanding. Though they remain committed to highlighting and exercising their work inside interactivity, they are limited by the singular theoretical model they perpetuate. At the same time, Milton Erickson and Carl Whitaker, among others, articulate no ideas about cybernetics while fully embodying it. With less concern for maintaining an unchanging model, their work was freer to change as their interactions with clients encouraged it.

Minuchin (1998) asked the field of family therapy where the family was in narrative and postmodern therapy. His question held the answer: there is no live interacting system in a therapeutic editorial or a postmodern reflection—only stories floating from afar. Yet the meta-story about the importance of stories, and especially the story about power dynamics, is dominant and reified in ways that are hyper-examples of the very agencies of domination from which many therapists invite us to seek liberation.

All clinical theoretical models and their accompanying pragmatic protocols are a set up for reifying an abstraction of choice (even if a therapist denies doing this) and then setting about to fix it. Therapists are either fixing problems (finding the right class of solution), family structures (a social chiropractic-like adjustment that realigns the family's hierarchical spine), patterns of interaction (disrupting sequences that hold irritating behavior), coalitions (undoing inappropriate alliances), social injustices (ignoring therapy and making it a populist education front for good citizenship), stories (beefing up overly thin stories or helping them be free from toxic cultural motifs), or the ever ubiquitous system itself (differentiating the social ego mass, fixing faulty communication patterns, and so forth). In all cases, the reified focus of attention maintains a particular model's definition of therapeutic reality. The client is implicitly asked to help the therapist verify the model. This is how therapy serves models rather than responsibly respecting, participating, and collaborating with the situational circumstances of people's lives.

ON NOT NARRATING THERAPY

One of the most important contributions to systemic therapy is the least mentioned today. Carl Whitaker (1976) proposed that theory, especially psychologically oriented explanation, was a hindrance to clinical practice. Adopting a Zen-like posture, he whacked the field with a wisdom stick, essentially saying that it was not about theory, interpretation, or grand narrative. It was about something that cannot be said. The relevant unsaid vaguely had to do with being in the here-and-now, but these words miss evoking the contextual complexity of experience that is moved by the particularities of relational engagement. Without freedom from the tyranny of any clinical model's theoretical interpretation, there is less chance for action born of the inspired moment, which is to say, inclusion in the circularities of each interactional turn of the ongoing performance. Though seldom uttering a cybernetic metaphor, Carl Whitaker's therapy perhaps best exemplified the shift from simple cybernetics to second-order cybernetics (see Keeney, 1983).

In addition to Whitaker (see Neill & Kniskern, 1982), there have been several therapeutic geniuses in therapy including Milton Erickson (see Haley, 1973) and Olga Silverstein (Keeney & Silverstein, 1986). None of them emphasized theory, explanation, or grandiose narratives. Their brilliance arose in the immediacy of interaction.

Following their example, we propose that there is no need for any form of reified Holy Grail in therapy—whether it be a system, cybernetic loop, dialogue, conversation, collaboration, reflection, neurolinguistic program, strategy, meta-model, narrative, gender role, or political agenda. Carl Whitaker is even more relevant today than he was decades ago: any importance given to a narrative, whether connoted as story or theory, hinders clinical work. When a story line and interpretation overrides experience, we lose touch and get out of synch with the circular interactions that generate the storytelling.

All narratives and theories potentially impede our being fully inside the circularities of existence. It is time to free the field of therapy from the sophomoric game of competing over who has the thickest conversation or biggest story. The latter only leads to the politics of banning certain metaphors, story lines, jokes, interventions, knowings, not-knowings, and ways of being alive. Let us be dedicated to at least mercilessly teasing all theories, narratives, and word games of therapy, doing so for the sake of being more improvisationally and therapeutically potent.

It's the distracting chatter that needs to stop. Ignore any dictum that sets up judgment of whether you need to listen or talk. Allow the situation to speak through you, whether it is through sound or silence.

It is time for another spark of creativity in a profession starved for imagination, freedom, and authenticity. Interact in order to be free from the totalitarianism of models and interpretation. Laugh about how passing a multiple-choice exam gives you a license to talk like a therapist. Ignore any simplistic moralism dictated by rule-governed models of practice. Love your enemy rather than maintain the premises of power that maintain the hatred. A transformation of hearts is better than rhetorical justice.

Note that our call to improvisationally act is not a literal request for the absence of theory, but is more an appeal for the freedom of theories to shapeshift as they appear, disappear, and transform. The hindrance of theory is more than a hindrance. It is a distracting irritation, a monstrous irrelevance, a tyrannosaurus hegemenous that has outlived its usefulness. Let us not weaken this liberating truth by saying you need to first learn the theories so you can later throw them away. The poets—and not the theorists—should be talking more. In their circling inside ever present paradoxes their words provide the best entry to the unspoken truths of empty stories ready to hold performed lives. It is time to act in ways that bring forth unspoken wisdom.

Any spoken theoretical narration must be set free as quickly as possible or else the string of words risk being presumed more solid than they are. As echoed in the Old Testament, you can't look back at any previously made interpretation or you risk being turned into a pillar of salt.

There is more than one way to relate to interpretation, narrative, theory, and understanding. For instance, whatever ideas and premises you believe are important will be subjected to endless paradoxical play and skilled interplay when you meet a Zen master, Bushman n/om-kxao (Keeney, 2010), experiential therapist, or Ericksonian inspired utilization-oriented therapist. They do not disagree that all the possible messed up things in the universe—whether it be brain chemistry, gender inequity, faulty family coalitions, limited life story, or traumatic childhood memories—may have given rise to the adaptive symptom you habituated to get on with your life. But they do not see liberation from this issue as derived from insight and understanding. The maestros of transformation work in the weave of the present interactions to utilize whatever arises in the systemic dance. Neither client nor therapist has to understand or preach about the reasons for things changing.

It is more likely that your fullest availability to being therapeutic will disappear when you serve a model of therapy rather than the mysteries of change. Therapy is a Zen koan: it has no answer that is right and is no more likely to solve life than theatre, religion, or weather. When we make therapy a game in which theory (or meta-theory) gets to sit in the throne, we all lose. The art of helping bring forth change asks us to go beyond theoretical discourse. It asks for its embodiment in ways that seldom need to be spoken except on those occasions in which it naturally expresses itself without preplanned intent or purpose.

If your therapy of tomorrow is the same as it is today, then your therapy is dying. Its particular form is only true for the moment in which it arose for the client who inspired it. In the changing of forms is found the wise process therapist, the practitioner of change who is always changing in order to help others change. Whereas first-order cybernetics asked us to take responsibility for changing the client, second-order cybernetics ups the ethical imperative by asking us to change ourselves in order to foster change in others.

The alternative to robotic therapies that are programmed by models is circular therapeutics - a changing therapist who is ready to be inspired by the movement inside each unique relational engagement. Little should be said about this to avoid risking another fixed position. It must be experienced and its appearance is dependent upon the growth of the therapist in more ways than can be articulated. All of us need a whack with a wisdom stick to help free us from the prison of any received view.

It matters not how many times you repeat saying or writing the word "system," "narrative," "postmodern," "interaction," "strategic," "race," "collaboration," feminist," "externalizing," "internalizing," "non-dualizing," "cybernetics," "therapy," "justice," "healing," "theory," "power," "mind," or "love." It is not the buzzword or name of the club in which you claim membership that is important. What is more worthy of our attention is how metaphors arise in the particular clinical situation that brings them forth. If you enter a session with know-it-all mind, you will act to verify the therapeutic reality in which you are pledged to maintaining membership. The alternative is "not knowing"—but not the feigned "not knowing" of a postmodern pluralism. We are speaking of a "not knowing" that is not interested in evaluating whether one is not knowing or not.

Post-model therapists are changing agents of change whose clinical experiences foster ever-expanding possibilities. They know not whether they will listen to stories or prescribe a ritual. They are perfectly comfortable seeing a social triangulation one moment, an attempted solution in the next, and a feminist issue at another time—or having none of these interpretations at other sessions. The liberated therapist isn't holding on to a list of therapeutic taboos or a code of banned, blacklisted forms of therapeutic understanding and action. Here you are free to be moved by whatever the client presents. The embodied circular loop of improvisation is the most respectful relationship possible with a client for it utilizes whatever the client and therapist bring and then utilizes what happens next in the interaction. We call this "circular therapeutics" and regard it as the key to bringing a healing heart to therapy.

It is time that therapists realize they are in the same domain of interaction as the Zen master and other interlocutors of transformation who mediate in the unknowing of fettered knowing. Let us become emancipated from being fenced in by any architect of an over-schooled approach. All schools of therapy are actually the same: prescriptions to follow someone else's arbitrary rules rather than being more flexibly responsive to what each session invites. This is a call to higher order ethics that is grounded in situatedness rather than a moralistic framework. As Varela (1999) notes, this is "a plea for a re-enchantment of wisdom, understood as non-intentional action." (p. 75) Here we find an invitation to be more creatively alive in a session and not be attached to any habit of thought or action that limits other possible ways of serving therapeutic transformation (Keeney, 2009).

Case Example: The Light Man

Court ordered therapy was conducted with an adolescent inside the walls of a state prison. Greg, a 17-year-old who had been incarcerated for nearly a year, was extremely emotionally upset and saw little hope in his life. With colleague Scott Shelby, we asked if anything had happened in the last couple of months that made him feel proud of himself. Greg replied that he had learned to make some minor electrical repairs and could remember the location of every light fixture he had installed in the prison. Immediately we asked, "Have you made yourself a business card for your future work? What would it say? What will you call yourself?"

Greg paused and then exclaimed with unexpected joy, "I got it. I will be the Light Man. I want to become the Light man. Call me and I'll install a light." Hearing his enthusiasm, a ritual was immediately inspired and prescribed: "We'd like for you to try a creative experiment tonight. Draw a light bulb on a piece of paper and when you've done that, write the name 'Light Man' inside the drawn bulb. Can you do this?"

"Yes, sir. That's easy. I like to draw."

"Tonight, before you go to sleep, place this light bulb under your pillow and sleep on it."

"Can I color it yellow?" he asked.

"Absolutely. Do just that and feel free to make any other interesting modifications," we replied.

The following week we found he had carried out his assignment and furthermore, had made a business card with two light bulbs drawn on the bottom at the corners. He also called his mom and told her he was the Light Man. Most important, he drew the image of a yellow light bulb and placed it under his pillow. To his amazement, Greg had a visionary dream:

> I dreamed I was in an aluminum fishing boat with an old wise man. We were in a swamp filled with alligators. While we were in the boat, I held a light for the old man to see the gators. The old man had grey hair and he had a friendly smile. Oh yeah, he was also wearing some alligator-skin boots. The man told me that he was gonna teach me some things. First thing he taught me was how to shoot an alligator with a crossbow. He also showed me his right hand and I could see his right index finger was missing. He told me that a gator bit it off when he was young, but that today he doesn't have any fear of them getting him. We talked about a lot of things. I was really surprised when he told me that he'd be back. He said, "I'll be back" then I woke up.

After hearing his dream, we encouraged the Light Man to draw an outline of a boat under his bed. "The boat you draw under the bed should be the same size as the bed. After you draw it, know that from this night on, your bed is never to be called a 'bed.' From now on, you must call your bed a 'boat.'"

Greg continued to have visions with the old man teaching him how to take care of himself and not be scared in the midst of dangerous gators and troubling situations. He learned that he could leave prison every night and visit the old man who he now called the Alligator Man. He told several inmates that he went to his boat at bedtime and that sometimes he received a sacred vision. That's when we told him to place his drawing inside a Bible and place it under his pillow. He replied, "That will supercharge everything."

His dreams changed from an alligator swamp to a recreational lake where he enjoyed water sports and making new friends. As these dreams changed, his life changed. He became a leader for others and helped them with their difficulties. He sometimes dreamed of them as well. One week, he drew another picture of a light bulb and invited us to sleep with it next to our beds. Yes, we each had a visionary dream that surprised us and encouraged our therapy to be even more of a mutual exploration of improvised experiments, encounters, conversations, tasks, performances, and transformations.

One of Greg's prison friends wrote a rap song that celebrated his life as the Light Man. We, in turn, were moved to provide him with our own spontaneous poetics: "The Light Man doesn't have to understand. He prefers making things grand. With his light he doesn't have to fight. His nighttime might make everything right."

Greg was released early from prison and he sent us a letter in which he said, "I hope the Alligator Man knows how much I appreciate what I learned from him while I was in prison. God is my light and I plan to bring the light to others!"

One more thing: we also made a videotape of some improvised blues music (Brad often plays piano in sessions) with lyrics about how a young man in a Louisiana prison had become the Light Man. We gave Greg a copy and told him that we were going to present it at an international brief therapy conference. He smiled and said, "Go spread the light. I know that my life is here for a reason. You know, we're in all of this together."

In this therapy we joined Greg inside a circular interaction that inspired us to improvisationally act without allegiance to any singular therapeutic model. Nor did any form of clinical understanding drive our action. We were not attached to interpreting and had no hegemonic commitment to maintaining any form of therapeutic propaganda. We didn't care whether it was systemic or not. Not did we once ponder whether we changed the class of solution, solved a problem, corrected a social coalition, worked with a narrative, voiced a postmodern sentiment, or moved around a cybernetic pattern. We didn't even ask whether it was circular. What we did was shaped by whatever outcome and communication Greg expressed. Without being directed by any school of therapy, we allowed the performance of our interactions to come forth in unpredictable ways that surprised and changed all of us. He dreamed and we did as well. In the turning of this embodied circle of relational theatre, he was set free from the tyranny of prison and we were able to escape the limitations of imprisoned therapy models.

Deleting Narrative

All models of therapy risk stalemating therapeutic possibilities when they dictate a template way of acting rather than being more flexible in dancing with each unique situation. Theories, models, meta-models, and grand narratives serve a useful purpose when they help free us from a previously stuck theory. Unfortunately, this new theory may then become the next ruling dictatorship that requires another theory to knock it off the block. This is true even for cybernetics unless we remember to activate its built-in escape mechanism, circularity, allowing a recursive re-entry into cybernetics that liberates any rigid theoretical attachment to its claims.

What frees us from being inside any theoretical-narrative-interpretive box and instead invites us to be part of an ever-changing circle of interactive performance? Try drawing a picture of a light bulb on a piece of paper and writing these words underneath it, "The Light Therapist." Place it under your pillow at night and then before going to sleep, try your best to imagine seeing the bulb lit up. Do so while not thinking about whether the words underneath your light mean that you should lighten up, become enlightened, or be someone who shines a different kind of light. If it helps, wonder whether it is possible to dream of being in a boat with an old character who will teach you how to quiet the snapping jaws of menacing alligators who say its all about the right words, stories, and understandings. Do your best to remember that a young man in a Louisiana swamp prison learned how to hold a light that helped him grow past his fears, worries, and impoverished situation. Maybe you will dream of him and hear him whisper into your ear, "We are in all of this together. Can I show you how to shoot a gator and light up the room?"

INTERLUDE

We once heard about a client who interrupted an important conference on psychotherapy. She simply stood up and asked a brief question, "Is therapy a poem?"

Silence struck the audience and the conference came to a halt infused with uncertainty. After a moment, an old man dressed in purple and sitting in a wheelchair, slowly raised his hand. With a twinkle in his eyes, he said, "I believe we have found a poem. Please tell me what you rhyme with?"

Not missing a beat, the client walked to the podium and took the microphone. After clearing her throat, she opened her mouth and pointed to the old man saying as slowly as anyone could possibly say, "I rhyme with you."

Leaning forward in his wheelchair, the old man replied, "Why of course you do. That's why what you say is true. It takes two to drop a shoe and spew a view that takes what's blue and cooks a stew for the very few who thought they knew how to construe a breakthrough that once upon a time grew a healing milieu."

3. Entering Interactivity: Steps to an Embodied Circularity

It may come as a surprise that the science of cybernetics provides a path to the heart of healing. Though often misunderstood and disqualified, it has always been concerned with the art and science of effective communication. What could be more applicable to our profession? It also addresses the nature of circularly organized processes that sustain life, whether found in the interactions of butterflies, families, clinical sessions, jazz bands, or redwood forests. This circularity is goal-oriented and self-correcting of its efforts to realize its goals, even at the level of maintaining the goal of maintaining existence itself. Cybernetics invites us to participate in the performance of circular therapeutics —being a circular participant interacting inside the circularities that organize our relational life, doing so to bring forth healing and transformative changes.

It is worth considering how cybernetics invites us to reframe our own profession's history. We certainly don't have to see this history as the evolutionary march from interactive system to individual interpretation portrayed by Hoffman (1993b, 2002) and Anderson (1997). What if we had a time machine and could go back in history, this time inviting a wiser handling of the differences that were being voiced in the field? We would then see more clearly how the key distinction of interactional circularity offered by cybernetics could have itself been utilized to engage in further critique and examination without losing sight of circularity and cybernetics altogether. Here offering (mis)interpretations of cybernetics would become less important than interacting with its metaphors inside the circular participation it invites.

Cybernetic participation could have organized and circulated inside the discourses that raised important concerns and considerations including feminism, social liberation, ecology, education, ethics, and all the rest. Without the primacy of interaction, we too easily drop the circular ball and run back to the old conventional way of bearing arms against the latest presumed adversary. The alternative is to stand tall and bring a relational and interactive wisdom that offers more than an either/or fight. Family therapy was once a custodian of systemic wisdom, but sold it out for a return to that which it had formerly liberated us from, doing so for reasons that future scholars will ponder. Was it because there was not a sufficient understanding of circular interactivity? Was it too difficult to teach therapists how to perform? Did some theorists not have the interactive chops to understand and enact what they were talking about? Was cybernetics itself entangled in muddles it had yet to clean up? Was Bateson only beginning to become the metalogue that performed his own circularity? Did the desire for clinical fame allow blind ambition to roll over wisdom and scholarship? Or was the seductive nature of a diabolical narrating mind responsible for putting a stop to more responsible action inside therapeutic drama, while claiming it was the moral enforcer?

The field saw a shining star, but it fell from the sky and the world went dark all over again. One model after another was propagandized as claiming the next truth, typically delivered inside a map of interpretation with a handful of clichéd lines of action. As the field became more lost, it became clearer that something was indeed lost. There was no longer wisdom nor extraordinary performance to guide it. Furthermore, it was disconnected to the healing traditions that had long addressed the ways in which healers can short circuit their work by listening to trickster stories, or becoming seduced by power, or following popular opinion rather than responsible leadership.

Our immediate mission is to recycle the important ideas that once had promise for birthing a competent and wise way of helping others with their suffering. We will return to cybernetics and give it a new re-entry. In subsequent chapters we will take this re-enchanted metaphor and carry it inside wisdom traditions that have expertise in quieting the narratives that trip us up and throw us out of tune. Let us begin again with cybernetics, this time asking therapists and cyberneticians alike to recognize that it can be regarded as more than an invitation to act: it asks us to act improvisationally.

CYBERNETICS IS IMPROVISATION

Cybernetics, when embodied in human performance and interaction, reveals the art of improvisation. By this we mean that a self-corrective circularity attends to how we utilize an outcome in order to improvise our next move, doing so to help accomplish our therapeutic goal.[1] In this circular therapeutics, a circle of interactivity invents each move in the ongoing flow of action. In improvisation no model, template, or map directs the action. It can change at any moment, dependent upon the outcome and opportunity at hand. As postmodernists Tyler and Tyler (1990, p. x-xi) argue, improvisation is "uninformed by 'knowing'" and is facilitated by "a being un-ready. . . in order to per-form without being in-formed." Here we find a model-free therapy in which the "therapist and client respond to one another without benefit of a script or even of a narrative." (Tyler et al., 1990, p. xi) Conversations do not follow a proper story line about pathology, whether it is localized inside psyche, family, or culture. Nor do they either ban or cling to particular expressions or forms of conversation in the name of non-pathology. Cybernetics throws us inside the crea-

---

[1] Recognizing that the word "goal" is attacked by some contemporary therapists as implying too much willful intent on the part of the therapist, we ask readers to consider whether they would want to be treated by a goal-less clinician who is even uncomfortable with hoping that clients are able to improve their lives. When an interpretation-focused therapist jumps all over a single term like "goal," "intervention," or "strategy" and protests every time they see it, rather than seeing how it is used and held inside a particular situation, they are behaving as a fundamentalist. This kind of dichotomous thinking is at the heart of our objection to model-driven, template-organized responses. They exhibit neither creative action nor critical thinking.

tive circle that does not reproduce the same form of therapy with each and every client a therapist meets. When one stops observing from a narrator's position—which is always disassociated from the stream of interaction—she is experientially transported to being inside the interactivity that was formerly distanced as the "observed other." Being inside interactivity is a "flow experience" that spontaneously moves all participants to bring one another forth.

Cybernetics is no stranger to the field of therapy, though as previously discussed, any distinctions it once offered, especially between "second-order" versus "first-order," have by and large been obscured, confounded, or misunderstood. It seems that the field is ripe for revisiting some of its ideas, this time as a way of preparing therapists to step inside a greater circularity of improvisational freedom. This is here where the heart of healing springs to life.

Whereas the last chapter sought to help liberate us from the domination of narrativity, interpreting, understanding, and self-verifying models, we now turn to throwing ourselves into interactivity, the circle that circulates ever-changing, relational co-invention, the construction of experiential realities that serve creative participation in life. Here narratives, interpretations, understanding, and models are spontaneously performed, but they are fleeting—present only for the situation that inspired them, and then let go. This is entry into the heart of healing, whether called the flow, the Tao, the mind of creation, the will of God, or the ecology of life. Cybernetics, as performance rather than interpretive lens, is an invitation to improvise life, another way of pointing to more liberated participation in the invention of our selves in relation to others.

Narrated versus Performed Cybernetics

Talking about cybernetics can be tricky, because doing so easily seduces us to sit in the narrating director's chair rather than be an actor performing on stage. The cybernetics of being an audience member (a first-order cybernetic production) joins us with the long lineage of desk-and-office-bound mapmakers who have simply turned cybernetic theory into another theoretical lens through which to construct interpretations and analyses. One can ask whether the latter provides an excuse for not taking responsibility for action—an evasion of ethics made possible by saying we should not influence or push ourselves inside a situation. A more seasoned ethical imperative declares that we are already part of the scene and cannot avoid stepping into the action. The cybernetics of performing on stage (a second-order cybernetic production) shines the spotlight on us and reveals how we are participating—whether we are fully present on stage or hiding in the audience.

Our present mission is to use cybernetics, and its distinction between first and second-order, as a means of tripping you to fall inside the circular interactivity of therapy. Here the difference between first and second-order should not be regarded as two separate cybernetic maps of meaning, or as viewing positions. It is about the choice of relationship you have with cybernetics: Is it a prescription for interactive inclusion or a description of a narrator's interpretative viewing? If you step onto the stage, the interactive play will move you. No map (theory, meaning, interpretation) is necessary when you are inside the moving flow of improvisation. Here interaction has its own mind and it has both higher order knowing and expression than that which is scripted by any previously constructed map or model. The mind of interactivity can voice itself through you, if you throw away your map and let the interaction speak. This is what it means for a healer to be an instrument of healing. Stepping inside the mind of a circle of interaction enables the emergence of transformation, steered by a relational ecology that is wiser than any preconceptions directing obedience to rigid protocol. The heart of healing arises when a therapist surrenders to circular therapeutics—higher order participation inside the living movement of circular interaction.

This is what Bateson was pointing to when he criticized purposeful behavior that was unaided by the self-corrective circuitry of more unconsciously held wisdom-mind. He warned against all simple models that claimed to have ready-made pat answers and action plans, whether pharmacologically driven psychiatry or pop psych models. Here the mindless administering of Prozac or a miracle question share a commonality—both are untempered by the deep circular wisdom that exists outside the range of a simplistic model. In the same way, the complex wisdom of Milton Erickson is lost when it is modeled and turned into a collection of strategies, routines, or clichéd utterances.

We are not arguing for any kind of fundamentalist return to cybernetics as an answer to our interpretive woes. Cybernetics is only useful to the degree to which we continuously interact with its ideas. That is, feeding cybernetics back into itself so that it may change as we change. After many years and visits to the epistemological crossroads since *Aesthetics of Change* (Keeney, 1983) was first published, we have found its truths are best conveyed through a more "poetic" handling of cybernetic metaphor. Cybernetics, as the formal science of circularity, must swallow itself to become reborn, here as the art of circular therapeutic performance. We suggest, however, that those looking for a detailed handling of cybernetics and therapy refer to *Aesthetics of Change,* cited by Heinz von Foerster (1987) as one of the classic texts in cybernetic theory. The ideas in this chapter (as well as this book generally) are not a departure from that work, but part of an ongoing, generative recursion of its ideas over the course of many years.

Another Round of First and Second Order

Heinz von Foerster (2003a) developed the idea of second order or "cybernetics of cybernetics," a term he credits to Margaret Mead. The distinction between first- and second-order cybernetics is one of the most important (and misunderstood) distinctions initially drawn within cybernetic thought. In the previous chapter we introduced it as involving the difference between interpretation and embodiment, or narrativity and interactivity. In other words, we are either describing a system's circularity from afar (interpretive narrating) or we are circulating ourselves inside the circularity we are interested in, whether it is specified or not (embodied interactivity).

First-order cybernetics is associated with the early days of cybernetic thinking when researchers described the circularity they perceived, but without explicitly making reference to the ways in which they themselves were in circular relationship with the observed system (Keeney, 1983). For example, a therapist might use cybernetic discourse to describe the circular patterns of interaction and feedback going on among members of a family, but fail to notice or remember that she herself is inside the circularity she observes, as she observes it. She observes and describes what is going on in a session or with a client as if she were outside or apart from both the interaction and her own descriptions of the interaction.

Now note the paradox that arises when we start moving toward a definition of second-order cybernetics: What is seldom mentioned is that a therapist can never be removed from an interactional circularity, though she may not recognize or make explicit that this is so. Her first-order cybernetic description—"I observe a circularity"—is generated from inside a circularity that is not mentioned inside the phrase, "I observe a circularity." However, the moment a therapist re-members her membership inside the circle, her first-order description explicitly re-enters the circling, birthing a so-called "second-order" circularity. Simply put, as soon as a therapist begins to interact with an individual client or family, her participation—which includes any observation, description, action, or communication she makes—is part of the circle of interaction that connects therapist and client. The recognition of this inclusion invites us to participate more freely and responsibly inside the circle of interaction from which we cannot extract ourselves, encouraging more improvisational acting. Therapists become free from searching for some underlying cause or uncovering more and more understanding before acting in order to know how to act again.

We can only become authentically collaborative, non-hegemonic, non-oppressive, relational, systemic, and mutually affirmative of one another if we surrender all our models and allow interactional movement to carry us more deeply into the circularities of relationship. A wonderful example of second-order inclusion lies in the masterful clinical work of Milton H. Erickson, whose practical emphasis on utilization points to the embodiment of circular interactivity. The alternative is to map the other, an act that keeps us separate (and hierarchical) from that which is mapped. All models ultimately disconnect us from one another as they impose rather than compose. Although they might be useful as training wheels for beginners, one must eventually become free of them and ride away.

The kind of therapeutic work called for in Anderson's (1997) so-called postmodern orientation is arguably more problematic than the models she criticizes. Unlike Erickson, she—and other orientations that share her sentiment—does not promote interactional expertise; it is banned. Note that Anderson (2007) also claims her approach is technique-free, but then prescribes how a therapist must act and communicate in order to be a dialogical conversation partner. These techniques include "jointly responding" through "reflecting, nodding, gazing, etc.", behaving so as to show that one is "being genuinely interested and curious about the client's story" and "pausing and allowing silences" (pp. 4-5). Saying that a therapist must take on the role of conversational partner itself limits therapists' choices of performance, including the choice to throw out all dialogical techniques.

At least interactional, strategic, and utilization approaches hold onto the most important dynamic of transformation—interactional know-how. The criticism of therapy models voiced by Bateson, and continued by Keeney, simply aimed to keep any circularity inside other orders of circularity. It was never about a retreat from interaction and a return to the psychoanalytic couch or conversational easy chair. Cybernetics, especially its re-entry into itself, helps free us to be more alive in therapy. It emancipates us from maps and the mapping that zaps creative opportunities for never-ending change. It does so as long as cybernetics is never frozen as a map, but remains a turning, changing circularity of circularity.

Be warned: cybernetics is not as complex as it may sometimes seem; it is also not as simple as it may appear. Cybernetics is most centrally about circularity. As Heinz von Foerster (1987) put it, "Should we name one central concept, a first principle, of cybernetics, it would be circularity."(p. 223) We take a first step toward complexity when we ask whether we are inside or outside a circularity as we discuss it. If we say we are inside a circularity, we immediately find that we must have been positioned as an outside observer in order to make that description (any "about it" commentary is made from the "outside"). Whereas a claim of being outside a circularity cannot remain true the moment we find that we are describing our relationship to a circularity, bringing us inside. Here the circularities of cybernetics breed paradox if we try to freeze our position as either inside or outside. If in, we are outside in order to say it, but if out, we are inside because it is we who are saying it. In other words, we are constantly moving around the circularity of observer and observed, self and other, as we participate in the interaction at hand.

Please know that if all this circular talk makes you dizzy, that's because you are moving with the discourse, spinning round its circular course. A circular therapist avoids getting stuck at a narrative or interpretive side stop. The alternative is to improvisationally act, interact, tinker and play in order to find yourself always circulated by the circle that does not require your commentary or understanding to keep turning. Be free to perform any kind of change and the circle will dance with you, reliable in its constant changing with each new turning.

One must be careful to not confuse the cyberneticians' inclusion of observing into the observed with Heisenberg's uncertainty principle. The latter laments how an observer interferes with making accurate physical measurements (measuring changes the measurement) and regards this situation as a problem and limitation that needs to be addressed. Cyberneticians, on the other hand, celebrate the inseparability of observing and the observed and invite exploration of how the observer acts in order to participate in the invention of the observed. Here we emphasize reality construction rather than its accurate representation. In therapy, we accept that the ways we act help bring forth both problems and solutions—or a universe where neither is relevant - in our clients. We take more responsibility for what we observe because we have a part in producing it. A therapist who does not act to change an impoverished situation is seen as an unethical part of the problem. As a therapist, you must change in order to become a part of the changing interaction and its transformed experiential reality.

Unfortunately, the well-worn distinction between a cybernetics of the observed system (first order) versus a cybernetics of observing systems (second order) led some therapists to think that the emphasis was upon observation, description making, interpretations, and map making. It would have been better for the original cyberneticians if they had distinguished between descriptive/explanatory cybernetics and participatory/embodied cybernetics. Descriptive and interpretive cybernetics—using cybernetic description as one observes, including the observing of one's observations—is different than embodied cybernetics. The latter enacts without having to enter any discourse that makes interpretive claims (Keeney & Keeney, 2012b). More important than having a well formed cybernetic description or interpretation is the performance of an un-formed (or even un-informed) improvisational presence guided by the recursions of interaction. RX: Let the maps go and become the territory.

Be Careful What Distinction You First Draw: It Will Come Back to Include You

G. Spencer-Brown (1969) distinguishes between the original act of creating an experiential world—the first making of a distinction—and its subsequent regress of indications, punctuations, framings, interpretations. The territory is found in the moving hand that draws a distinction, while the map emerges in the recalling of that distinction through all the indications and names we ascribe to it. For therapists, primary acts of distinction set a reality in motion that is self-verified by ceaseless re-indicating. If you distinguish a problem, any discourse about it—whether aimed at interrupting its habituated pattern, searching for solutions, or re-authoring its story—can have the same effect of maintaining its indication. That is, it keeps the problem alive and on center stage.

Practically speaking, if a client reports that a problem or issue won't go away, we can assume that there is a circular pattern of organization that holds this experience—it recycles its appearance. Of course, the client is inside this circle as are all relevant participants who interact in the scenario. When systemically oriented therapists propose that symptoms are held inside a pattern of interaction, they are pointing to circularly organized systems that go round and round without the desired correction. Whether demarcated as cognitive loops, problem and attempted solution interaction, or choreographed family coalitions, these circular patterns are vicious circles that maintain an ongoing replay of the drama.

It is important to remember that the circularity of therapy includes a therapist maintaining the role of a client. As Bateson (personal communication with B. Keeney, 1996) once said, "Therapy involves proving the difference between who is the therapist and who is the patient." Healing moves past therapy by taking away the therapist's scripts, models, and maps that prescribe being a therapist. A healer paradoxically surrenders all expertise to be empty—actually more empty of knowing than the client—and invites the client to perform inside the circularity of interaction that draws upon greater wisdom than any role-prescribed means to therapeutic ends. Here we may be tempted to say that healing is about proving there is no difference between therapist and client.

If an initial distinction is made to establish a difference in relationship, all subsequent performance will act to construe the priority of this difference. When prisons are built, people in trouble with the law are gathered and given further instruction in how to be criminals. Build it and they will come: distinguish a context and it will automatically bring forth its own membership. Similarly, therapy can be a contextual trap that teaches people how to be professional clients. Be careful of the distinctions you draw for they will come back and not only include you; they can become you.

From *Circulus Vitiosus* to *Circulus Creativus*

Circularity in the context of human interaction illumines the familiar dynamic of the "circulus vitiosus" or vicious circle (von Foerster, 2003b, p. 230). A basic, popular example is one in which a person might describe being caught in a vicious circle with regard to overeating: a client feeling discouraged about his heavy weight responds by eating in order to reduce the discouragement, which then creates yet more feelings of discouragement over having eaten too much, to which one responds by eating more, and so on. There might also be any number of vicious circles operating in the therapist's relationship to his practice. Sometimes the more a therapist tries to be spontaneously creative, the more clichéd his actions seem, and then the more exasperated he becomes trying so hard to be creative, the more contrived and non-spontaneously he performs.

One of the great Occam's razors in the history of therapy was the idea of problem-solution interaction advanced by Watzlawick, Weakland, and Fisch (1974). Here a problem is regarded as maintained inside a circular interaction with attempted solutions. Problems do not exist unless there are attempted solutions keeping them on stage. The Watzlawick team's therapeutic strategy is to change the class or type of solution. For example, a client with speech phobia can announce his fear of speaking at the beginning of a speech rather than try to alleviate it. This surrender to the problem sends the attempted solutions home. In so doing, the problem disappears.

What is overlooked when this idea becomes a model of therapy is that all solutions, no matter what their class, may contribute to perpetuating some class of problem. The very idea of solution keeps one mindful of the problems that are needed to prove it is actually a solution. Here we start to enter a second-order circularity when we expose how the problem solving therapy approach itself may be an attempted solution that is invested in the existence of problems to maintain its presence as a professional activity that can relate to them.

Similarly, there is no escape from a problem focus when we turn matters upside down and say we are solution focused. From a second-order perspective, solution focused and problem focused therapies are the same: both are examples of problem-solution (or solution-problem) interaction. Looking at exceptions and future miracles is as likely to maintain the hunt for exceptional problems and future disasters that are required to prove the veracity of their twin counterpoints. Might someone ask whether a miracle for therapy would be to imagine a future without either problem or solution focused therapists? After all, searching for either a problem or solution constructs a home for both.

Therapists may easily become stuck in a vicious circle that maintains a model rather than serves transformative change. However, rather than lament the circularities that maintain trouble for both clients and therapists, we join Heinz von Foerster (2003b) in suggesting the liberation of circulus vitiosus from its "bad reputation," raising it "to the honorable position of a circulus creativus, a creative cycle" (p. 230). Healing includes the transformation of vicious circles into virtuous circles. Said differently (and more cybernetically), circular therapeutics welcomes our being inventors of new ways of performing inside our patterns of interaction, releasing ourselves into the freedom that comes with the creative play of circularity. This requires less sideline interpretation, pathologizing, psychologizing, and systemic viewing of individual or family behaviors. Adding explanation or so-called understanding does little to lift us out of the vicious cycles in which we experience being caught. Healing transformation instead calls for creatively acting and interacting in new ways so as to tinker and experiment to create differences that can make a transformative difference.

The utilization of a problem, remarkably exemplified by Milton Erickson's clinical work, demonstrates how a problem changes when it is made an ally rather than an enemy. This implicit second-order know-how allows a behavior to change in a stream of ongoing interactivity rather than be highlighted and fixed by our efforts to eradicate it. Whitaker's psychotherapy of the absurd follows this tradition of working with the problem rather than fighting it. One does so not to trick the problem into being solved, but in respecting that there is more to a problem than what appears problematic. It enters the scene with something to offer, whether connoted as a teaching, a metaphorical communication, or a co-therapist pointing the direction of change.

Externalizing a problem or claiming that the problem is the problem contributes to problem saturated discourse. Worse, if the problem is ridiculed, scolded, or attacked, the systemic weave that holds its presence is fractionated and reduced to another dualism that is even more ready to perpetuate suffering in other life challenges. Imagine telling an alcoholic to swear at her addiction rather than accept that she has no power over it, the latter being the wisdom way that AA prescribes in order to paradoxically handle the double bind bred by mind-body dualisms.

One more time: if we second order a therapy, we turn it on itself. The problem eradication of problem-solving therapy requires liberating it from an over-attachment to only seeing problems and attempted solutions as the organizing distinction. There are other circularities of interaction in the world that can be spun, including the distinctions of over-seriousness and attempted humor, hopelessness and attempted inspiration, boredom and attempted living. A second-order solution focused therapy might look into a crystal ball and see the ultimate solution of no imagined solutions or miracles. Here life is what it is, without unnecessary connotations that distract from being in the here and now. This, of course, does not mean an absence of change, but change that moves along naturally without the roadside stops that look for solution mirages. Finally, narrative therapy enters its second ordering when its story becomes thick and complex and recursive enough to include a main character, perhaps a therapist, whose life is not organized by stories.

When circular therapeutics invites us to second order our relationship with clients, we find that their problems are their solutions, our diagnosing is our intervening, their therapy is our therapy, and we are both solved when we interact unrestrained by a model, map, or theory. Old-fashioned therapists used to say that such therapy is alive, enabling both therapist and client to be nurtured and grown. Old-school healers say that healing heals both healer and client—there is not one without the other. In the second ordering, the therapist-client interaction treats the client-therapist interaction. More abstractly, a circle circulates its own circularity.

Therapy should be more than an entanglement with problems and solutions. It should be more like a tango that helps us all find virtuosity. With a healing heart, each session serves the creation of virtuous circles. This can be accomplished by focusing on the strengths and resources of a client and therapist (rather than their solutions) or by transforming a vicious cycle into one that moves toward virtuosity. We participate in the latter when we creatively interact with a so-called problem, rather than going into combat with it. It is more collaborative to collaborate with problems, and it is just as collaborative to collaborate with strengths that are equally present in the communications a client brings to a session.

SELF-REFERENCE IN THERAPY

Because there is always a circularity between describer and description, there is no description, theory, map, model, or interpretation that does not reference or contain the observer who puts it forth. Cybernetics challenges "objectivity" in a unique way, placing a circle around object and subject so that their interaction is seen to circulate, relate, and interpenetrate any of their assumed differences. Said more poetically, we are each recursively poured into the unfolding of every moment such that however we frame or punctuate our living contains our living of it; our process of knowing is inside our action as our action brings forth our process of knowing.

Heinz von Foerster (2003c) once said, "...tell me how the universe came about, and I will tell you who you are." (p. 293) Likewise, when a therapist describes a client, he tells you what kind of therapist he is. A resistant client is inseparable from a resistant therapist, even if the latter is only resistant to resistance. If a therapist is made anxious by a client's anxiety, prescribing an anti-anxiety medication for the client helps the therapist's anxiety subside. The therapist might as well have taken the pill himself. In the early days of family therapy, some family therapists only prescribed medication if the whole family agreed to take it. Similarly, if the family insisted that one member be hospitalized, the whole family got checked in.

While cybernetic self-reference dispels the idea that any kind of "objective" observation is possible, it goes past arguments for the inclusion of "the subjective." The recursive self-reference of cybernetics is meant, as a description, to render the mind's dualism of objective/subjective moot. It is intended to bring us into the performance of the "not one, not two" paradox of Zen, helping us escape our reification of what is certainly a felt human experience of there being an inside/outside, subjective/objective split. In a metalogue entitled, "What is an Instinct?", Bateson (1972) expresses it this way:

Daughter: Daddy, are animals objective?
Father: I don't know—probably not. I don't think they are subjective, either. I don't think they are split that way. (p. 48)

Too often the cybernetic notion of circular self-reference never gets past a clichéd repetition of "everything said is said by an observer" (Maturana & Varela, 1980, p. xxii). In both therapy practice and pedagogy, this is often reduced to the invitation to reflect upon and analyze ourselves as observers, and then construct various interpretations about how this impacts our work with clients. It has been suggested, for example, that supervision in therapy programs should include an emphasis on continuous reflection and discussion about how trainees' personal backgrounds, assumptions, and social identities shape the way they listen to and interpret what a client presents. This orientation trivializes the more cybernetic invitation to leap into creative, improvisational interactivity that reinvents one another.

Constructing narratives and interpretations of our selves (and our clients) outside the therapeutic interaction eclipses and even restricts both therapists' and clients' capacity for unpredictable change. This includes the way a client's experience and communication may not "fit" whatever list of characteristics we were told they would in our cultural competency course or in McGoldrick, Giordano, & Garcia-Preto's (2005) book of ethnic stereotypes. Hermeneutic self-reflection is an ineffective approach to interrupting any tendency on the part of the therapist to ignore his or her own biases, overlook human difference, or miss the complexities of social interaction. This is because interpretations are always partial and biased, and when generated outside the interaction of a therapy session, they easily become fixed theories, ideas, stereotypes, and distorted lenses that then shape our therapy, even when the intention is otherwise. This is as true for stereotypes that suggest "all women are passive" as it is for a stereotype that suggests "all women suffer the effects of the stereotype that all women are passive." The latter, though in some ways created to challenge the former, generates yet another stereotyped way of relating to clients.

Reifying a therapist's reductive interpretations about her own experience—such as her belief that because she is a woman this makes her more likely to be sensitive to relational dynamics among clients—perpetuates the processes that generate arbitrary human categorization (e.g., definitions of race, gender, ethnicity, class, etc.). Similarly, if a therapist says, "As a man I am aware that clients who are women may find it difficult to trust me because of the dynamics of inequality and violence perpetuated by patriarchy, so I must work to build trust," he is making assumptions about how his clients who are women will relate to him before they even walk into the room. When therapists are instead guided by the circular interactivity in a session, the interaction itself will be the compass, not any well-meaning critical consciousness about the dynamics of oppression. Inside the stream of interaction, any awareness the therapist has about the ways in which gender differences are able to make a difference will not impose themselves before they are interactionally called forth for examination. We should avoid all preconceived generalizations that discriminate before we have even been introduced to the client.

In summary, beware of constructing a reference library that catalogues and categorizes narratives about the self. This is the same process that generates categorical knowing about another. The cybernetic idea of self-reference simply means the therapist and client are always encircled inside continuous change, the ongoing movement of which is inseparable from their participation. Here inseparability is paradoxically freeing; it frees us from referencing and clinging to any story, narrative, or interpretation to instead be guided by the movement of interactivity in a session. No understanding of the past or present is necessary. Let circularity, not preconceived understanding, be your guide. When you jump inside the circling of circular therapeutics, you and the client have all you need in order to kick-start innumerable possibilities for creative change.

THE PARADOX OF CIRCULAR AUTONOMY: CLOSURE OPENS INTERACTIVITY

After so much description of circular interrelatedness, the word "autonomy" may seem like a contradiction given its pop-psychology connotations of self-sufficiency and independence. We will see, however, that it is the circularity of relations that generates autonomy. Consider how a circle's geometrical form is closed—there is no opening. This closure gives it autonomy or distinctiveness from its surrounding medium. Cybernetically speaking, the "closure" of circularity in a system's organization is the very form of description that allows a system to be identified as a system, both distinguished from and capable of being-in-interaction with an environment.

For second-order cyberneticians, there exists a kind of paradoxical openness from closure where "a system is open to its environment in proportion to the complexity of its closure" (Clarke & Hansen, 2009, p. 7). In other words, the more organizationally closed a circularity, the more interactivity it can perform. It is organizational closure that creates interactional openness. A well-circulated mind is not closed-minded; it is organizationally complex in its circuitous pathways, enabling more openness to diverse thinking. For example, fundamentalist thinkers cannot interact with a wide variety of ideas. They must keep their world leveraged on the dualism of a simple right versus wrong. Though we often refer to this as closed mindedness, from the perspective of circularity, it indicates weak organizational closure that cannot compensate for too many variant perturbations, irritations, and challenges. A more closed, complexly organized circularity can handle divergent encounters and is therefore more interactive; that is, it can participate in a wider range of conversations, dialogues, challenges, creative productions, and invention. The same holds true for therapists—model-driven therapists are less interactive/generative/creative than the more organizationally closed, or autonomous, improvisationalists.

Again, it is impossible to not be inside a circle, for however long and in whatever situation. The question here for therapists is what circle organizes you in a clinical session. When the closed circle entails a therapist inside a model of therapy, all a therapist can do is self-verify the reality of the model. Again, the client is there to help the therapist prove that the model is true. Circularity, with its utilization of difference that drives improvisation, is banned. Instead, parroted, pattered, non-interactive responsivity is mindlessly exercised. A religious fundamentalist will say that if you do not subscribe to his or her exact beliefs, then you are against God. The only acceptable set of responses is "you are saved" or "you are lost." Similarly, there are therapists who claim that if you do not practice a particular orientation, then you are against collaboration, solutions, or sensitivity to cultural or other differences in life experience. But we all know that if a therapy model does not talk about chocolate, this does not mean that its proponents dislike or disregard the existence of chocolate.

If the circle is the interaction of therapist and client without constraint by a model, anything can happen. A new therapy can be invented for each session. Of course, there are always constraints operating on the interaction, including the desire of both to achieve a successful outcome. What is most important is whether the circle of interaction primarily serves transformation or verification of a modeled reality.

Organizational closure reminds us that not only is the whole never simply the sum of its parts, there is nothing going into it that gets processed and then spit out. There is no funnel into a therapist's mind into which we can pour clinical knowledge. Nor is there any tidbit of understanding or technique that can be taught and later tested. Among other things, this means that the multiple-choice licensing exam is trivial. It either shows that a therapist has been made predictable and independent of interactivity, or as is more likely the case, it only demonstrates that a therapist is obedient to an organization that demands that she momentarily perform trivial responses in order to receive permission to practice.

Models of therapy perpetuate the same kind of predictability as licensing exams. They prescribe correct answers, understandings, and actions, doing so as if they apply to all situations. All models act as if diverse contexts do not exist. They run against the grain of embodied interactivity, inspiring trivial participation that often succumbs to boredom and malaise in the session and the profession. The big choice for therapists is whether they step inside the circle of a therapeutic model's way of reproducing its self-verifying tenets or whether they step inside an un-informed per-formed interaction with each client, allowing something to be collaboratively improvised, invented, and created. The former exploits the client no matter whether the model makes a claim to be liberating, collaborative, or therapeutic. The latter utilizes both client and therapist, offering them to a circularity that can surprise and change both.

What circle will you step inside? Do you belong to a circle of like-minded therapists who celebrate membership in a common way of organizing sessions so that it verifies the veracity of a school of therapy? Or do you join each client in a newborn circle that is free to create interactions that are liberated from clichéd responses? The heart of healing, circular therapeutics, serves the circle of each particular moment. It views licensing exams and schools of therapy as the productions of disembodied practitioners. Therapy moves toward healing when a greater circularity utilizes the participation and contributions of both client and therapist to be more than they are in their separateness and their distinct roles. In this circle, both are renewed and revitalized as improvised participants inside creative transformation.

CASE EXAMPLE: SELLING A CANCER

Brad was conducting a demonstration session for an audience of mental health workers in Canada when a middle-aged woman from the audience interrupted his session. She shouted out, "Stop! Please stop. I need to talk. I cannot wait any longer. I am sick with cancer and need to work with you now." Her request was both sincere and desperate. He started talking to her as she sat in the audience. What follows is a transcription of their session. Here is an example of conversation that is not guided by any model of therapy. Each response is improvised and steered by the circularity of interaction holding the encounter.

The session demonstrates how interactivity alone can steer therapy, without any allegiance to a model. Of course, there are basic premises associated with interactivity that are inherent in transformative work. They include commitment to utilization, emphasis on resourcefulness, collaboration with the interaction (rather than with an individualized therapist or client), and a heartfelt desire for the client and therapist to help one another affirm and celebrate the mystery and beauty of being alive.

Brad Keeney: I need to ask whether you live in an apartment or a house.

Mary: I have a house.

BK: Does it have one floor or two floors?

M: Two floors.

BK: I'm speaking to your unconscious. What floor does that part that you worry about live on?

M: It lives in the basement.

BK: The basement. Which corner? Or is it a corner? Or is it in the middle? Is it in a box? Is it wrapped up? Has it been forgotten?

M: It's funny. I see two places. I see the bedroom, and I see the basement. In the basement I see it over in a corner where the laundry area is.

BK: Is it wrapped in an old newspaper?

M: Well, as soon as you say that, I see that.

BK: Is it a classified ad?

M: Well, it could be. I'll go with that. I see the print. It's black print.

BK: What might it say? What might one word be in that print?

M: The space of time.

BK: Perhaps you are looking at a classified ad. At least you've seen it as such. For a moment, this thing is wrapped in old print with words giving it a particular meaning. Maybe you should think of putting it in another room.

M: It's kind of horrible. I don't really like it. It's kind of like a hard turd or something.

BK: Yeah? Well maybe you should give it a makeover. *(They both started laughing.)* What I was thinking of when you first spoke is that somehow it's good for you to move your furniture around in your house. When was the last time you changed your furniture, I mean, moved your furniture?

M: Well, just a week ago, I brought a piano in. My father died recently, and my parent's home has just been sold, so there's been a lot of furniture moving. I have been selling and letting some things go. There's a whole family structure that's now gone. I brought the piano in. I was going to sell it, but I brought it to my home, and there're only certain ways the furniture will fit because it's a small house.

At this point, Brad felt it was time to bring Mary to the stage. Prior to this they had been talking back and forth across the audience. Brad asks her, "Would you mind sitting up here?"

After Mary came up and sat down, Brad turned away from her and gazed at the place where she had been sitting the moment before. He pointed there and started a talk that brought what they just said to the present moment.

> BK: You know the last time I was here, there was a woman sitting over there who reminded me of you. She had a similar complaint.
> M: Hmmm.
> BK: She was worried about her life, about something that had come into her life, into her body, and didn't know how to relate to it and was confused about the choices. She didn't know whether to see it as a disease that threatened her life or to see it differently. Many people made suggestions, and she was frustrated about how to sort through all of that. As best as I can remember, I asked her where she lived. Did she live in an apartment, or did she live in a house?
> M: Right.
> BK: She said, "A house." I replied, "Was it one story or two stories?" She answered, "Two stories." And I said, "Where in that house did that surprise guest reside?" She then said, "I think in the basement." For some reason I asked, "Is it wrapped in old newspaper?" She answered, "Since you asked, I can see that." And then I asked her, "Is it classified, a classified ad?" Members of the audience laughed when I said that. I wasn't sure why they laughed. I was confused by their laughter because I was exposing classified information. So I thought to myself, I wonder what she would see, because she was so focused and serious about this matter. I was sure she would take the next step and put a little effort into trying to bring her inner focus to help her see what was written on the newspaper. She saw the single word "the."

M: Oh my God!

BK: Then she said there were some other words. They were either the space of time or the time of space. I thought to myself, well that covers it all: space and time, time and space. Add an e to the word the, and it becomes thee. Eternity.

M: Yes.

BK: I remembered that the day before the woman had asked me, "Could we have a chance to talk the next day?" *(Mary had asked Brad to have a session the day before, though she said nothing about her condition.)*

M: Which I did.

BK: I was awakened in the middle of the night with the idea that I would speak to you later that day and that I should tell you that you should move your furniture around. Being a very different kind of person, I no longer have any curiosity as to why I would dream such a thought. I just know that I will say it to you and that it is the right thing to say.

M: Of course.

BK: I just remembered to remember that thought for that space and time. So at this time and in this space I think it might be interesting for you to know, like that woman *(Brad looked to where she had been sitting)*, and this woman *(Brad looked at her)*, there's always at least two floors.

(Mary nodded her head in agreement.)

BK: Sometimes you can go up, and sometimes you can go down. But for all the things in your house, you do have some say about where they're going to reside.

M: I do.

BK: You can give them different names. Sometimes you can worry about them. Sometimes you can laugh about them. Sometimes you can even—That's it! Oh, I just got a little ripple of excitement. This is what I think you must do: you should put a classified ad in the newspaper seeing if anybody would like to buy this part of you.

(Mary immediately burst into laughter.)
BK: The ad should say: "My cancer's for sale."

As Mary gasped and laughed from her belly, Brad shouted out, "Whoa, isn't that an interesting way to live!"

Someone in the audience shouted out, "Wonderful!"

BK: So you'll have to decide.
M: I'll have to decide.
BK: You'll have to decide how big the ad will be.
M: And which newspaper it will go into.
BK: You just might consider a full-page ad.
M: All right.
BK: It depends on how important it is for you to get on with this.
M: Right.
BK: But of course, you know, if you see a full-page ad, you can always reduce it to being a small full-page ad that will appear to be a smaller ad although it's actually a full-page ad in your mind because that's how it began. These are important choices, but only you can navigate through that. You can know whether it's going to be small or big. Whether you'll describe what you're offering as small or big, and of course, whether it's small or big depends on what floor it's on and how it's staged to the world . . . Will your ad say, "For sale: A part of me"?

Someone in the audience provided another way of advertising: "Do you want a piece of me!" This brought a lot of laughter.

BK: Some might propose, "Cancer looking for another home." . . . Is it going to be for free? Or are you giving it away?
M: No.
BK: Some ads say that a person has something and they are looking for somebody who'd like to take it.

M: That's true. I just did that with my parents' furniture.

BK: You could have a yard sale.

M: *(Mary nearly fell out of her chair laughing, but then turned serious.)* Okay, I can see that, but somebody picking it up bothers me. If I make a newspaper ad and put the cancer for sale along with some of the old knickknacks of my folks, someone will come around and ask, "Oh, what's this? I'll buy it." I don't want somebody taking that.

BK: Oh, so you prefer keeping it in your home.

M: No! But I don't want somebody else taking it into their life.

BK: Then you'll have to change it so it's something that you will be happy to see them take . . .Why don't you say it's a pet cancer? Maybe you need to put it in a birdcage. What kind of cage would you choose? Would it be a cage for hamsters or a cage for . . .

M: I saw a birdcage.

BK: What size?

M: I saw one of those old-fashioned birdcages.

BK: Yeah, that's what I saw. Victorian?

M: Yes.

BK: That's what I saw too. Interesting. We're in the same space and time, aren't we?

M: We're in the same space and time.

BK: Would it be—

M: It might be hard to give away!

BK: That's what I was thinking! Maybe you'll decide that this cancer should be your pet held in a cage that makes it beautiful. I don't know! Maybe you just need to move it around first. Put an ad in the paper saying you're thinking about giving it away and you'll entertain offers. Or maybe you should go halfway in between. Maybe you should rent your pet cancer. People could check it out for a couple of days.

M: No! None of that! I know about teetering around with it. I know about how it can come and go. Yes. No. Yes. No. Here it's back. No, it's not. Oh, I'm healed. No, I'm not. Oh, I know about the vanishing and reappearing act.

BK: You know about being inside a cage.

M: Absolutely! Absolutely! *(She started to weep.)* I do, though it has brought me so many gifts. But I still can't get it out. I know the shadow of it. I know the shadow of how it has defined me. I know the shadow of how it has been my—

BK: I know the word. It has been your master. You've been the pet. It's time to turn that around. Go get a cage of the right size for the right space so you'll see who's the master.

M: I will do that.

BK: And put out an ad.

M: I will do both.

BK: Great!

M: I previously asked for a dream in case we would meet and talk about my situation. I had two dreams. Do we have time for me to speak about those dreams?

BK: Yes, it's always time—

M: And space.

BK: This is the space.

M: A number of months ago, I had a dream that I was in a room and there was a woman behind the desk. She had her magical objects in front of her. I couldn't see her face.

BK: This is what we've been talking about, you know.

M: Yes. And there were boxes like bento boxes on the desk. I then saw an image of myself, and I said, "That isn't for me anymore, but this image is. I can pass over to another image of myself."

BK: We've been talking about this today.

M: Yes, exactly. In the next moment, a young woman from my high school who I haven't thought of in a long time suddenly appeared. The woman behind the desk said, "Ah, she knows everything about benches, and she will find your bench for you. I'm going to make a ceremony for you. The tumor is over." After that dream I had a lot of difficulty. My father died, and he had always been working with me.

Furthermore, the tumor that had been contained for about three years has grown. It has grown over the last few months, which has been upsetting in terms of what that might mean. I feel that the dream hasn't come to completion and there's something in me that is not able to complete—

BK: Well of course! It's because you're out to lunch. *(They both laughed as Mary got the joke.)*

M: Yes, you mean my bento box. *(A bento box is a Japanese lunchbox filled with all kinds of savory surprises.)*

BK: Then maybe you need a bench. It would be a nice place for that Victorian cage which holds all your old-fashioned ideas.

Mary literally rose from her chair, and her whole body trembled from head to toe. She exclaimed, "Oh! Love that!"

Brad pointed to her body and shouted, "Oh yes! That's exactly what you should do on your bench. That is it!" Brad pointed to how she was shaking, and he demonstrably shook to add an emphasis to the importance of her ecstatic body expression.

BK: Do this so you can move around all the furniture within you.

The audience shouted, "Yes! Yes!"

What was remarkable about Mary's dream is that the ancient samurai healing practice that is part of Brad's training is called seiki jutsu. It refers to the art of moving the life force throughout your body, doing so for healing and well-being. When this takes place, you can see your body tremble, shake, and make automatic movements. Its practice takes place on a bench called a seiki bench. Mary's dream and her trembling body held all this wisdom. Brad enthusiastically praised these aspects of her report, including her reference to Japan with the mention of a bento box.

BK: You know what to do. So go be it. In this time and space. For all space and all time, and any time and any space, first or second floor.

Even in a basement. Inside and outside, do it for her. *(Brad pointed to where she had been sitting in the audience.)* She was like you in a time I remember not so long ago. Because that time is this time and all time.

Metaphorically speaking, on one floor, things appear, while on another floor they disappear. Each floor is a different place and time, a separate reality. We are free to move from floor to floor, shifting from one reality to another, doing so as we watch former things vanish while discovering other things come to life. On one floor, we're inside a cage; on another, we are free. In one space, it's another time. In another time, it's a different space. Her ideas about her cancer were free to move in any direction and be as small or as large as she chose.

Brad received a letter from Mary several months after our session. She wrote:

Hi Brad,

I wanted to give you an update. I posted an ad in the *Toronto Star* entitled, "Cancer for Sale—no longer have time or space." I found the perfect birdcage in a drive by sale on the way to a cottage. I also sent the cancer a "Dear John" letter. I actually mailed it. I think it was sad, but understood it was over. The furniture in my house is moved.

I went to the corner of my basement and found I had stored a painting there that I did not like because of an abstract shape in the corner of the painting. It was sitting where I said the cancer lived in my house. The painting is moved. Perhaps I will leave it somewhere fitting in the city.

The shift from fear to confidence around the cancer was dynamic from the time we worked together. Thank you.

I recently received a checkup from my surgeon. Although the tumor was still there, the horrific surgical side effects she had previously discussed with me as a 50-50 risk factor had changed to being negligible. She also let it slip out that I would live to be an old lady. This comment could not have been based in her reality of talking to a patient with recurring cancer, but it was mysteriously said anyway. I felt my life had shifted into a new dimension of reality.

My longing is to keep the shaking happening and to keep on going.

Shaking all over,
Mary

Several months later she sent another letter:

Greetings Brad,
I met with a friend yesterday who I have not seen in years. She told me she had heard of someone who had placed an ad in the paper to sell their cancer.
Living in a new way. I will be in touch again.
Big love and delight to you,
Mary

Interlude

Did you hear about the therapist who rented a hot air balloon? He wanted to travel to heaven and ask God for a healing heart. In his balloon, he climbed higher and higher into the air. Then he stopped climbing. He leveled off and soon began to sink. Assuming he was as close to God as he ever had been before, he looked straight up and shouted to the sky above, "If you are listening, please tell me how to climb higher and reach you."

To his surprise and to all those on the ground below, the sound of a lion's roar was heard, followed by a road sign that magically floated in midair. It said, "Keep asking and leave an offering."

The therapist never stopped asking how to climb higher. Every time he asked, he made an offering. When he ran out of all his material possessions, he offered each and every one of his ideas, beliefs, theories, and understandings. He did this until he was empty inside and out. That is when he started going all the way up.

Just before he reached heaven, a messenger flew up to him with a message written on a tiny strip of paper. It said, "You need three things in order to learn that there is only one thing. Go home and find them."

4. Holding Interactivity: A Batesonian Tool Kit

Let's circle back to the distinction between therapy and healing. Are they two or is one inside the other? Is healing the heart of therapy? Or does therapy with a heart of circular interactivity bring forth healing? Does a healing heart bring a therapy of therapy and the healing of a therapist? Does healing require a heart that is free of therapy? Is there anything that can be said to help us become wise, creative performers inside the circles of therapeutic transformation? Is circular therapeutics found in the never ending circulation of circular interaction?

When we shift to an emphasis on embodiment, the observer moves past observing, including observing observing. Here we surrender to the interactivity inside an improvising circularity. Though scholars have argued for the differentiation between distinction (I/it; observer/observed) and embodiment (I/Thou; relata/relata), there has existed a conceptual blind spot where it is not seen that this distinction itself does not necessarily help achieve embodied embodiment, creative creation, participatory participation, and therapeutic therapy.

The leap into circular inclusion is vitally important. What begs closer attention is an examination of what is involved in making the shift to circular therapeutics. Truly moving to an inclusionary circular epistemology is more than the stuff of description, ideas, or even particular actions; it is a kind of leap into another world, a leap made difficult by the fact that what we see will always be shaped by the world in which we are presently operating.

There is a tendency in the space of transition to understand or perceive another way of punctuating our reality, but to then reduce or collapse this new way of operating into the same old epistemological premise—it is possible to describe what it means to be out of the box while never leaving the box. Leaving the box (or making the leap) has been described as moving from lineal to circular causality, reproductive modeling to transformative process, fragmented to interpenetrating ways of knowing reality, and therapeutic narrating to interactivity. Getting to the latter side of the distinction, however it is named, requires both a new order of distinctions and a way of handling them that is improvisationally guided to create differences that make/create/invent ongoing differences.

A BATESONIAN HANDLING OF CIRCULARITY

The way in which Gregory Bateson drew upon cybernetics and circularity, formerly called "Batesonian epistemology" (Keeney, 2007, p. 884), offers us a circular way of handling circularity. It is comprised of three conceptual "tools" that are useful in helping us more effectively embody circular therapeutics: (1) logical typing; (2) the nature of difference; and (3) recursion. As tools they serve as another way of further illustrating and elaborating the descriptions of circularity presented earlier. They shed additional light on the transformative implications of circularity for therapy, in particular the levels of difference involved in stepping from circular description to circular performance. Here we find another way to point toward what is involved in awakening a healing heart for therapy.

There have always been therapists who are allergic to theorizing and prefer emphasizing that they are more experiential, process oriented, in the here and now, intuitive, and complex. However, saying this does not mean that they are. At the same time some therapists claim to follow a specific orientation or model of practice, but are actually improvising in the here and now. Bateson's conceptual tool kit helps us bridge the gap between narration and performance, enabling us to have a way of talking and explaining that serves our being inside the flow of interactivity.

LOGICAL TYPES. Bateson (1972) was fond of applying logicians Whitehead and Russell's (1910) theory of logical types to communication to keep track of the level of abstraction used in a discourse. In particular, he emphasized distinguishing between the level of abstraction called "context" and the level of abstraction concerning particular actions. For example, therapy is the name of a context whereas a client's smile refers to a simple action. Distinguishing ("typing") the different levels of abstraction in the way we describe a phenomena was a critical tool for Bateson, providing a way of uncovering how, in our everyday handling of language, we create different orders of distinction and then mix them up, thereby producing both the best and worst of human experience.

When Virginia Satir helped clients (and therapists) differentiate between descriptions they have of sensory experience versus their hypothesis about what is going on inside a person, she was implicitly utilizing the theory of logical types. You can see a "smile," but you cannot see "happiness." The latter is what she called "mind-reading" another person's state of being (Satir, 1988). It is the name of the context that gives meaning to an action, but it is not directly perceived. One could be smiling to cover up pain or employing a tactic that helps sell an idea. When a smile is typed by an observer in a way that pleases the person smiling, that person feels "seen," but if the smile is mistyped in an unpleasant fashion, there is an experience of relational disconnection. If I wink and you correctly name the name of that action as a "flirtation," I am pleased if that was my intention, but embarrassed if it belonged to the context called "clowning around."

Bateson illustrated this distinguishing of abstraction through his often-cited reminder that "a name is not the thing named" (Bateson, 1972, p. 280). Eating the menu (the name of the food is a different order of abstraction than the food) may provide a moment of comic relief in a Marx Brother's skit, but it is regarded as a matter of schizophrenia when done in the context of a restaurant where nutrition is sought.

Human beings constantly mix up logical levels and this shaking up of abstraction underlies schizophrenia, many kinds of suffering, but also humor and creativity. Eating a menu gets laughs for a comedian, but diagnosis for a mental patient.

Therapists as well produce their own form of professional schizophrenia and suffering when they mix up abstractions, especially those reifications that mystify and constrain rather than clarify and liberate. The very act of placing a particular adjective in front of the word "therapy" and then claiming it as a distinct model sets up a crazy message that other therapies either do not include or perhaps even oppose that which the adjective is being used to describe or indicate. Brian Stagoll (2000) makes a similar point in his criticism of "narrative therapy." He questions what makes it so different from other forms when "all psychotherapies are based on 'narrative', going right back to [Freud's] Anna O, and the 'talking cure'. . . To speak of Narrative Therapists is a bit like talking of Heart Cardiologists, or Shoe Cobblers, or Systemic Cyberneticians." (p. 124)

We could say the same about "behavior therapy," "cognitive therapy" or "emotion focused therapy," for after all what therapy does not face behavior, cognition, and emotion? On the one hand, these adjectives help others know what is emphasized in the therapy model. But this kind of naming has the political consequence of staking a territory in a way that implies they, and not others, are giving adequate attention to that chosen metaphor. This is particularly the case with a name like "Just Therapy" and other therapies that go out of their way to highlight that their model is concerned about oppression, justice, and liberation. The implication is that therapists who choose not to follow these schools are either not critically aware of social problems or do not care about or act for justice and greater equality. The result is that self-ascribed liberation therapists who desire freedom and equality arbitrarily impose a border around both therapists and clients who do not talk their particular talk.

Paradoxically, we often find that people become the opposite enactment of the metaphor they advocate. Hence, peacekeepers and defense programs sometimes perpetuate conflict and war while freedom fighters advocating peace start fighting an enemy. Similarly, "just therapists" can perpetuate an oppressive form of justice talk, systemic therapists can become lineal propagandists of systemic reductionism, narrative therapists can fail to ever restory their narrative about therapy, and postmodern therapists can too easily become modernists in their attachment to an absolute truth that says no absolute truths exist. This kind of outcome typically arises when we are bound inside a particular class of theory, ideology, or therapy school, while implying that other nonmembers are distinct from the name that is used to name our class or type of orientation.

A more commonly recognized way of indicating the different orders of description immanent in the ways we communicate is Korzybski's (1994) reminder that "the map is not the territory" (p. 58). [Though at a higher order of circularity, the map *is* the territory, as von Foerster reminds us.] It should be no surprise that the literary master of playing with different orders of abstraction was Lewis Carroll, whose work Bateson often cited as a demonstration of how we construct worlds that create havoc when levels of abstraction are confused in unexpected ways. In Alice's world, the song, "Haddock's Eyes," is not the name of the song but the name of the name of the song (Bateson, 1972). One might curiously muse and possibly confuse the world of therapy by asking an Alice-in-Wonderland-like question as to whether a problem is the name of the problem, or the name of the name of the problem? Does this question concern problem naming or the naming of problems, or is there a difference? If so, is this the difference that matters when it comes to problems and their naming, or transforming problems named?

Another way Bateson's thinking is relevant to therapy is exemplified by Keeney's (2007) exposition on the ways of knowing in the spiritual experiences of the Ju/'hoansi Bushmen of southern Africa. He uses Batesonian epistemology to unmask the encompassing "contextual weave" that holds different orders of abstraction involved in describing/knowing diverse aspects of Kalahari ecstatic healing, such as a particular action (e.g., "trembling hands") versus its larger context (e.g. , "healing") (p. 886):

> Logical typing also helps us distinguish "healing" as a name of contextual organization rather than regarding it as a name of simple action. For the Bushmen, the simple actions inside a context of healing include trembling hands and bodies, singing, clapping, tightened abdominal muscles, and shrieking sounds. None of these actions in themselves defines healing. Healing comprises the more encompassing pattern that weaves and choreographs the various actions into a context that facilitates transformational experience. (p. 885)

Applying this form of analysis to transforming therapy, we can distinguish the different levels of abstraction associated with particular actions or behaviors in a session (e.g., complementing a client, identifying a solution, interrupting a sequence), and the more encompassing context of a session as "transformative," "creative" or "healing." The presence of particular actions or behaviors commonly associated with progressive, alternative, or creative therapies does not necessarily constitute or indicate the more encompassing transformative contextual organization of one's practice.

Simply asking a "miracle question," for example, is submitted as proof that solution-focused therapy has been performed. Or that giving a paradoxical homework assignment indicates the practice of strategic therapy. Unfortunately, therapy models end up operationalizing their approaches into simple actions like these, enabling them to fit into an empirical research study and thereby qualify as a member of an evidence-based class. They do so at the cost of becoming reduced to a collection of trivial actions and meaningless clichés, rather than a masterful weave that changes as change enters the scene.

Finding a healing heart for therapy requires more than reproducing simple actions and claiming they are indicators of a class of therapy. Praying with a client, asking them to discuss spiritual topics, wearing Tibetan beads, or saying "Amen" does not assure that it is a context of healing. Nor does saying that you are a healer or have an awakened heart. Healing, like therapy, is a name of contextual organization. If you are in a healing context, everything you do is healing, including reading the phone book. If you are not in a healing context, nothing you do is healing, including reading a sacred book.

A healing context arises when interactivity is moved by orders of process and transformation that are held inside an ecology of wisdom. Little can be said about the latter for whatever is said is only a slice of its whole complexity. Suffice it to say that we know when a context is healing by how it feels when we are in it, assuming we are tuned to notice it. Entry into healing includes being inspired by the uniqueness each situation offers. This requires our being more committed to the contextual organization of therapy rather than any simple action that purports to indicate a particular methodological orientation. Specifically, healing asks for a heart-centered context that inspires relational interactivity, giving rise to actions that turn the circle of interactional circularity—a circular therapeutics. Anything less risks our becoming a cog in a trivial machine that has no heart or soul, performed mindlessly on an unlit stage silent of co-participatory performance.

THE NATURE OF DIFFERENCE. Bateson's proposal of a second tool ("the nature of difference") is actually inseparable from the first tool ("logical typing"). Distinguishing logical types or different levels of abstraction in our making of description is a natural consequence of our understanding and exercising the nature of difference. When we act upon George Spencer-Brown's (1969) proposal to draw a distinction in order to create a world, we remind ourselves that our acts of creating bring forth the differences that distinguish a world.

If a therapist asks a client to describe the problem, construction of a problem-centered context commences. On the other hand, inquiry about the last tasty dessert a client remembers marks a turn toward exploring delightful experiences in life. Even if a client says, "I am suffering," a therapist can respond, "I am impressed by how you said that. Your speech conveys passion and conviction. Have others told you that you have a distinctive way of talking?" Now the session focuses on competency rather than deficiency. The indications we make contribute to the therapeutic reality that is constructed in each session.

Be careful to not naively assume that there should be a ban against metaphors about problems, suffering, or bad times. Sometimes we may feel compelled to utilize a focus on symptomatic occurrence or problem solving, but we do so freed from any model that stereotypically dictates how to handle our discourse and experience. What matters is whether interactional circularity moves and comes to life. A lively and creative encounter with problems is better than a stereotyped boring discussion of solutions, resources, or positive living. Utilize whatever has creative life in a session. If a client complains that his or her everyday is dominated by the problem, you might be inspired to comment that the problem may be lonely for another problem. Ask the client what kind of other problem would be a good friend to the singular problem. Of course, this should only be done if this direction spontaneously arises in a live session.

Bateson, like other colleagues who subscribed to a radical constructivist orientation and found George Spencer-Brown's work to be foundational (Keeney, 1977, interview with Bateson), wanted to underscore the act of creating when we distinguish. This is more than an inclusion of the observer's participation in observing. It is emphasizing the act of invention in the prescriptions for descriptions of observing. In one of Bateson's (1972) well-known examples he suggests that Newton invented, rather than discovered, gravity. Similarly, problems and solutions, as well as therapy and healing, are invented. This is not to say that people do not suffer or that therapists do not help, or that objects do not stay on the ground. It is perhaps wiser to say that we invent the ways we distinguish suffering from healing and the ways we interact with both, and knowing this gives us more choice of action. The more we can generate different ways to face the situations clients bring to us, the more likely we won't get stuck in any one way of working.

Therapists can benefit from revealing and highlighting the initial acts that give rise to a therapeutic reality. A critical examination of the observing system, which may be oneself, is intended to spotlight the primary acts of distinction that bring forth a reality, rather than offer a retreat into the kind of self-inquiry that looks like the historical analysis of one's psychological and sociological traits and circumstances. The shift to a second-order cybernetics of observing systems aims to show how the observer's observations were created by acts of distinction rather than interpretive maps. These acts are the things said and done with a client, not the unspoken biases and beliefs inside the therapist's way of understanding. Again, we see how the ways we acted in a session brought forth our understanding rather than introspect over how our understanding steered our interpretive reflections. As Heinz von Foerster's (2003a) work asserted, the shift to emphasizing the presence of the observer in the observed (or the therapist in the therapy) brings us more responsibly into the ethics and aesthetics of how we interact with others. It is an ethics/aesthetics of active invention rather than passive reflection.

When Spencer-Brown (1969), a protégé of Bertrand Russell, launched his *Laws of Form* while a professor at Oxford University, he formalized how the foundation of mathematical thinking and logic itself could be understood by tracing how distinctions distinguish themselves in patterned and embodied forms. While his work removed the need for logical typing as an injunction banning paradox, Bateson's use of logical typing was not to ban paradox, but to keep track of how different orders of abstraction are utilized to construct descriptions and experiential realities. It enables us to say that no simple action is in itself a context, and this includes both therapy and healing. Again, it is nonsense when a school of therapy makes a list of simple actions and claims that this operationally defines its therapy. It is no more than a pile of actions that when added together only makes a pile, not a contextual weave. It takes a weave of action, woven by the movements of interactivity, to spin a context. If a pile of actions is dumped in front of a client, independent of their having been produced in real-time interaction, there is no therapy. Such action is not essentially different than leaving a therapy textbook on the client's front porch.

If a client has been manipulated to play along in the reproduction of a previously designed ideology, orientation, or therapeutic model, then we have the trivial learning that is like the multiple-choice quiz. Obedience rather than transformation takes place. This is true for all schooled therapies. They trivialize and reduce the possibilities for creative action because no therapist is wholly present in the room with a client. They are tracing the outlines of a map rather than exploring new territory.

It is sheer nonsense to claim a collaborative therapy if the latter follows the same set of rules and procedures for each session. The client is stuck fitting into the therapist's orientation. It is the same if the therapist naively thinks the client knows how to proceed and then sits passively waiting for direction from the client. It is clients' interactivity, rather than their individuality, that should organize therapy. Any professed postmodern therapy should appear improvisational and not be informed by any preferred way of thinking or acting. Otherwise, it is an imposter. Finally, any claim to be a liberation therapy is a farce if it frames liberation in a way the therapist dictates. Therapists must stop eating their menus and asking their clients to do the same. The alternative is sharing a meal and enabling everyone present to be nourished.

It is important to note that Bateson was more than concerned with distinguishing the difference between a simple action and its contextual organization. He required that we develop our abilities to be both keen observers of action and thinkers with clear abstractions, skillfully handling metaphors that are appropriate for an indicated domain of experience. Therapists have to guard against the temptation to think that context (and especially the abstractions that indicate it) is more important, thereby implying that any close observation of action can be made secondary or irrelevant. Perhaps Bateson's finest contribution was his prodigious ability to observe action. The same was true of Milton Erickson whose work builds upon finely tuned observational skills. After all, utilizing requires perceiving what can be utilized.

Some therapists, thinking therapy is all about interpretation or story, lose sight of the importance of observation. It is not atypical for them to remove themselves from the clinic and to prefer writing letters to their clients, given the primacy they give to textuality and storying. Therapy that is driven by interaction, collaboration, and participation requires experiencing the client with as little drift time into introspective hypothesizing as possible. Otherwise, a talking head may only observe its talking head observing.

Another clinical mishap of logical mistyping is frequently found when clinical supervision takes place in the form of discussing a case or watching a videotape. This often reveals a supervisor who is not handling the difference between narrativity and interactivity. Video review is "dead supervision," a postmortem analysis of a session after it was alive. Though a post-hoc exam may be interesting, it teaches narration and interpretation about an already performed therapy. When interactional and systemic therapists claim that clinical video reviews are superior to live supervision, as we once heard a former director of a systemically oriented institute proclaim, it is an indication that they are teaching interactional viewing rather than interactional doing. Only live supervision provides a real-time opportunity to teach how to be inside the weave of an ongoing interaction.

RECURSION. Bateson's final tool, "recursion," is itself derived from considering how the nature of difference can circularly operate on itself. Drawing a distinction leads to distinguishing that distinction and on and on one may go distinguishing, that is, indicating without end. The dynamic of distinguishing, the ongoing re-entry of distinguishing distinction, is recursion, the circularity that operates upon itself, embodying the circling that creates circularity. Recursion is not repetition, but circular re-entry with the utilization and production of a different order of circularity.

Jung (1974) was aware of the importance of recursion when he discussed the alchemical symbol of Ouroboros:

> The alchemists, who in their own way knew more about the nature of the individuation process than we moderns do, expressed this paradox through the symbol of the Ouroboros, the snake that eats its own tail. The Ouroboros has been said to have a meaning of infinity or wholeness. In the age-old image of the Ouroboros lies the thought of devouring oneself and turning oneself into a circulatory process, for it was clear to the more astute alchemists that the prima materia of the art was man himself. The Ouroboros is a dramatic symbol for the integration and assimilation of the opposite, i.e. of the shadow. This 'feed-back' process is at the same time a symbol of immortality, since it is said of the Ouroboros that he slays himself and brings himself to life, fertilizes himself and gives birth to himself. He symbolizes the One, who proceeds from the clash of opposites, and he therefore constitutes the secret of the prima material . . . (para. 513)

Von Foerster and the founders of cybernetics were all fond of using

Ouroboros as a symbol for their primary idea of circularity and its more processual and embodied form: recursion. Devouring distinction and turning distinction into a circulatory process is the *modus operandi* of how realities are constructed. This includes the making of our own identities, as Jung noted: "devouring oneself and turning oneself into a circulatory process." It is also true for creating a therapy with a healing heart: it requires devouring therapy and turning therapy into a circulatory process. Circular therapeutics invites us to leap from being a collection of models to being an inventive recursive process where interactivity is moved by improvised circularity.

Note that the three conceptual tools presented by Bateson are actually only three ways of describing one tool – the circulatory process of recursion. Each previously described tool is an enactment, or an unfolding in time, of recursion. Bateson's tools—logical typing, distinction, and recursion—are one and the same tool, but expressed at different orders of abstraction as each act of distinguishing a tool leads to the next tool. An example: Noting that the therapist is not the therapy (tool 1: *different logical types/levels of abstraction*), we may note that our noting is the act of drawing a distinction (tool 2: *nature of difference*), which in turn, enables us to see the circularity inherent in distinguishing "therapy," that is, we distinguish our distinguishing of therapy (tool 3: *recursion*). The paradox is that at the first order of abstraction, the therapist and therapy are separate, whereas at the highest order of recursion, the therapist is the therapy. The middle level of abstraction – the act of drawing a distinction – is the fulcrum, the point where both possibilities (domains of knowing) reside.

This unfolding of distinction, the turning of Ouroboros so that it generates different orders of abstraction/description/knowing/bringing forth, constitutes creativity. The alternative is to engage in reproduction or template stamping: stamping everything with the same mold, map, model, grand narrative, or set of distinctions. It is not even enough to say that our tool has the name of recursion. We must recursively generate, create, and bring forth recursion so that it may be realized in never-ending operations, enactments, and embodiments.

Embodied circular performance aims to create, invent, and bring itself forth each time it takes the stage. It does so without knowing what will appear until the circling action of distinction and emergent differences begin to dance. Different orders breed surprise, confusion, contradiction, ambiguity, and all the other necessary conditions for the complexity that serves the creation of the creative process. When a therapist empties her narrations, throws away all models and maps, and jumps into the circularity of improvisational interaction, she finds that a session creatively wakes up. This is not a plunge into chaos and reckless action (even if it is, there is more to what is going on than the limitations this evaluation implies.) Any ecosystem, from an inland lake to a clinical conversation, is self-organizing and self-correcting. Leave an ecosystem alone and it regenerates itself. This was a teaching of Gregory Bateson, who argued that the forest has a mind that is more complex than the limited circularities of our individual minds. The wisdom traditions ask that we attune ourselves to be in synch with the greater mind, the circularities that are weaving us anyway, whether we resist or cooperate. When we are a cooperating "part of" this more complex weave and effortlessly move with it, our hearts soar like an eagle. That's when we know healing has entered the room.

Keeney (1983) once proposed that the art of therapy was giving the illusion of doing something, while actually doing nothing. But this not doing is a higher order doing, a performance inspired and moved by interactions that include the contributions and participation of others, inside and outside the clinic. The greater circular mind of therapy holds the wisdom that steers change. Again, when we follow it, or dance with it, our heart is awakened and healing emerges as we become inseparable from it.

Making the Leap into Circularity

In Zen Buddhism, paradoxical encounters are sometimes used as tools for liberating stuck habits of distinguishing. As Bateson (1972) suggests, finding oneself in a context in which one's previous ways of distinguishing and acting no longer "work" or make sense is what holds the potential for sparking non-trivial change in one's way of knowing. He offered this example from

Zen: A master tells his student, "If you say this stick is real, I will strike you with it. If you say this stick is not real, I will strike you with it. If you don't say anything, I will strike you with it" (Bateson, 1972, p. 208). Here the master has removed all possibilities for logical response. For any resourceful transformation to occur as a result, the student must creatively jump outside the box. Hence the intentional use of the double bind in Zen as a means of bringing forth "enlightenment," or a mind of no limits "...in which personal identity merges into all the processes of relationship in some vast ecology or aesthetics of cosmic interaction." (Bateson, 1972, p. 306)

Bateson (1972) claimed this kind of learning or transformation "is likely to be difficult and rare even in human beings" (p. 301). It points beyond the ability to describe circularity, nonduality, enlightenment, or even to distinguish between different types of learning and contextual punctuation. The latter refers to how we habitually frame contexts and thereby organize our action. A higher order change involves a radical transformation of punctuation itself, liberating us from framing, as interaction alone self-generates contextual diversity. The latter dissolves any fixed narrative steering of a performance in favor of interactivity's ceaseless participation in the acts of creation.

Again, and it can't be said enough, we must be careful to notice that though our viewpoints may change or multiply, the essential premise producing them may remain the same. The mental health professions typically become more skilled at inventing new punctuations with the same premise of distinction – more models are proliferated of the same logical type.

We draw the parallel of the Zen master who discerns the difference between a student who can describe the non-dual awareness expressed through the words of a koan, versus one who embodies and performs non-dual wisdom: "As generation upon generation of Zen teachers have stated, it is a mistake to think that one can solve a koan merely by analyzing it intellectually" (Loori, 2006, p. 127), that is, by finding the right interpretation or understanding. The same is true for "solving" or "resolving" the contraries and complexities of life in a therapy session.

Bateson (1972) reminds us that "there are always loopholes by which the impact of contradiction can be reduced" (p. 303). In other words, the mind is tricky and when presented with paradox, it will often quickly collapse into more manageable dualisms, even while it may still be able to describe the present paradox. This process underscores the way therapists might be able to describe some version of second-order cybernetics without ever embodying or performing the circularity a true entry into second-order cybernetics brings. Saying, for example, that you "embrace paradox and ambiguity" or "circular epistemology" in your therapy or worldview carries a certain intellectual currency in the field of therapy, but its discursive repetition alone lacks the epistemological "oomph" of a good koanic double bind held inside real-time interaction.

The leap into circularity is always a recursive one. First-order cybernetics need not be thrown away in order to embrace second-order cybernetics. Second order takes place when a first-order circularity recursively operates on itself. One doesn't walk away from circularity; one feeds the circle to itself in an Ouroborean way. The latter is recursion and it requires a first-order circle in order to have a second-order meal. Though it appears that first order has disappeared when you swallow it, it is now inside the second-order circling, embodied rather than separated as distinct. It is there even when it isn't.

Similarly, the therapist must throw away therapy in order to embody it. There is a partial truth to the invitation to stop being a therapist for therapeutic reasons. This paradoxical recursion spins you into the heart of healing. Here we find that there never was a leap from our starting point. There is no need to abandon or negate the point at which we begin. What is needed is circular movement that acts upon itself. An entry into circular change finds you becoming constantly turned by ever-changing forms of change. This is where anything said seems contradictory and paradoxical as the saying changes its point as it continues saying. Change in order to find yourself. Hold onto the beginning in order to reach the end. Walk a straight path in order to return home. Welcome to a circularly organized poetics that silences cybernetics in order to voice its circularities.

From Cybernetics to Healing

We would be very happy if we never ever said another word about cybernetics. We say this for cybernetic reasons. Our wish is to embody its circular wisdom and create expression that is the enactment of its paradigmatically different way of being in the world. To only write about it and offer another understanding in the game of theory-making eventually becomes boring and lifeless. We feel the same about all theory and reflection that sits still and does not interact with itself in ways that bring forth the possibility of dismissing or silencing its textual stasis.

During the 1960's Rollo May invited Gregory Bateson to a gathering of humanistic psychologists in Tucson, Arizona. Bateson surprised and likely irritated his audience by proposing that there was no paradigmatic difference between humanistic and behaviorist psychology. All models of psychology, he argued, belonged to the same materialist paradigm that had no relationship to the importance of pattern, circularity, or the "reasons of the heart."

Family therapy, especially systemic family therapy, once claimed to be an alternative paradigm to all of psychology. It even called itself a revolution in mental health. But today we see it is time for a Batesonian sentiment to again be expressed: there are no paradigmatic differences found in any of the therapy models. They all freeze-frame experience into a static template that neither points to circularity nor circulates in any embodied practice or expression. Systemic therapy and narrative therapy, structural family therapy and feminist therapy, strategic therapy and Bowenian therapy, and all the other models, are more alike than different. They are members of the same class of paradigm, residing next door to the psychological models that were built before them. The way out of the paradigm of boxed-in therapies is to leave the more encompassing box form that holds them all. Outside its boundary is found fresh air, the breeze of a revolution that awaits us in each and every clinical session.

Let us not forget that there have always been and always will be therapists who step outside the mold and dare to be free therapists, thinking and acting freely as the interactivity of every unique situation calls them to be. Whether known or unknown, these model-free therapists are alive and well as they embody less in-formed and more per-formed ways of being. Pause for a moment and listen to the beat of the drum inside your chest. It is announcing a march that will lead you outside the Box of boxes. Detox your box practice, and take the first step toward the door. Hear the metaphors it rhapsodically sings – utilization, improvisation, circularity, interactivity, heart, and the poetics of circular therapeutics. Utilizing improvisation, circularizing interactivity, rhapsodizing the heart, we dance inside the poetics of a circular therapeutics.

Hence, we call for the circular embodiment of healing that frees us from cybernetic interpretation and any other narrative, theory, or paradigm that implicitly suggests faithful allegiance. We wish to dance with what cybernetics has inspired and to interact with its implications so as to give rebirth to the truths it articulates whenever it desires to have another say. Later in his life, Heinz von Foerster essentially called for the same, saying that cybernetics had less currency the moment more people assumed they knew what it meant. This very critique enabled Heinz to emphasize again that it is not the knowing, interpretation, and understanding that are primary. It is the way we are prompted, inspired, and moved to act that matters. We regard this movement away from a theory of cybernetics to a poetic performance as a liberating creative recursion. It sets us free to be inside the circle of creation rather than an outside postmortem commentator who endlessly drivels on as if speaking about a corpse stretched out in an examination room.

The move from therapy to healing requires the same leap of action. Neither a specific understanding nor particular faith is required. Simply act in order to know that there is more than knowing involved when one participates in healing interactions. A healer is not a born-again cybernetician. Healing is the never-ending birthing of whatever the cybernetic, circular processes that organize our living happen to bring forth. A healer moves with the "bringing forths" found in the heart of interaction.

CASE EXAMPLE:
THE GREEN LIGHT

This case example introduces some lessons about a therapist accessing the resources he has that can awaken his healing heart. Here the case itself is the teaching and no commentary is necessary. As in all of our work, interactivity alone guides it. Whatever emerges is circulated and embedded within other circularities, doing so to weave a context that facilitates transformation, all done without the purposeful hand of intention. This is unschooled therapy; a way of collaborating with the client that utilizes whatever comes up and allows it to move us into new territory where there are no maps. We allow healing to arise and ride along with it. In this case some important teachings emerge that can help all therapists find their healing heart.

Jim is a therapist in his sixties who lives in a small town in the Midwest. He has had a successful career developing and directing social service programs. Faced with a promotion that would require that he and his wife of forty years move from their large home out in the country to a condo in the city, Jim has begun to think about where he'd like to retire and what kind of life he would like to live as he gets older. Jim isn't exactly sure what he wants to "work on" with us, but he indicates feeling "stuck," and that he "intuitively" knows now would be a good time to seek out some new inspiration.

Note: The first thing that happened in the session was that Jim dropped his cell phone on the floor upon entering the room. Oddly enough, the wallpaper picture on the phone changed to a photo of a bright sun. Jim noted how strange that was because he had never seen that photo before.

Jim begins the session by telling us a little bit about himself.

"Well, I love to fish. My wife, Beatrice, and I moved out to this beautiful home in the country many years ago because we both love all the lakes. She loves to paint. She is an artist. I would fish while she painted the landscape."

We asked Jim if he and his wife ever thought of painting a beautiful mural of a country lake scene on the wall if it turns out they have to move to the city.

"Oh yes, actually Beatrice has painted murals in our home here. And right now she is actually out in New Mexico staying with our son for a few weeks while she paints murals in the grandkids' bedrooms."

Brad asks, "Jim, if your wife were going to paint something very unusual on the wall in your new home, perhaps something that no one has ever seen before, what would it be?" Jim thinks for several minutes, in silence.

"I don't know," he says. "I can't think of anything." We end the first session with the first directive:

"Jim, the next time you talk to your wife, I'd like you to think about this together. If you were going to paint something unexpected or unusual in a mural on a wall in your home, what would it be? Just enjoy talking about it and don't be too concerned with coming up with a good answer. You might come up with several. Just allow yourselves to dream about that a little, perhaps even allow yourselves to suggest absurd things that you would never imagine painting on a wall. It doesn't matter, but just make sure you have that conversation. Can you do that, Jim?"

Jim agrees that he will have a discussion with his wife.

"Another thing," Brad says. "Next time you come see us, I'd like you to bring a paintbrush with you."

"A paintbrush?"

"Yes. Don't worry about what it means. I'm not even sure why I'm asking you to bring one; it just popped into my head."

"Okay," Jim chuckles a little, "I suppose I can ask Beatrice if I can borrow one of her paintbrushes."

"Great."

***

A few weeks later Jim returns. He hands us a paintbrush with a green handle. We thank him and put it on the table in front of us. We ask him for a report on the conversation he had with Beatrice. "Oh, I actually forgot to talk with her about it," Jim replies. Before he can say more, Brad interrupts:

"Jim, what is the strangest thing that has ever happened to you?" Jim thinks for a moment, and says, "Oh, I know. Something strange did happen once, many years ago."

He immediately begins sharing a story that occurred more than thirty years ago. He and his wife were living in a town that had a large Mormon population. One night their son, still a baby at the time, had fallen ill and two Mormon missionaries happened to knock on their door. Realizing Jim and Beatrice had a sick child, the Mormon couple asked if they could come in and pray over him. Though not very religious, Jim and Beatrice thought it good to accept this offer and so handed their son to the couple to hold. Then something very strange happened:

"All of a sudden, while they were praying over our son, I looked over near the fireplace and saw two glowing green lights. They were like two small figures a few feet high, one a bit taller than the other, but not well-defined, sort of like glowing blobs of green light. Beatrice saw them too."

"And then what happened?" We asked.

"Well, the Mormons also saw the lights and got very scared and immediately gave us back our son and left. That's all I remember." Jim goes on to tell us that he doesn't really "believe in things like that," and that if it hadn't happened to him, he never would have believed a story like that.

"But it happened," he said. "Beatrice and I are not into that sort of thing. I mean I don't even know what it was. And I'm not saying it *was* anything, but... well we saw it, both of us. And so did the Mormons. It was strange."

We immediately express our wonderment at this story.

"What do you think it was?" we ask.

"I have no idea. It wasn't scary, though. It was just kind of strange. It made us feel good. It gave us a tingling feeling over our hearts. It was a good thing. I do know that."

"So who else have you told this story to?" Brad asks.

"No one, actually. I think I may have told one or two close friends. But we don't really talk about it much."

"Really? So you and Beatrice, how often do you talk about it together?"

"Never, really."

"When was the last time you talked about that night?"

"Hmm. Gee I can't remember. It's been years, I'm sure. Yeah, we don't really talk about it."

We continue to celebrate the extraordinary nature of his experience with "the green light" while remarking on how interesting it is that he and his wife never discuss it.

"You know, Jim, there are lots of people who would just love to experience something like that. I don't know what it is either, but clearly you had a very special encounter with something mysterious. And it happened while people were praying for the healing of your son. A lot of people wouldn't be able to wait to tell everyone about it, but you and your wife basically never discuss it. That is quite interesting." Hillary says.

"Yes, my sister is that way," Jim explains, "interested in spiritual stuff, I mean. We don't really get along. But she is into all that supernatural stuff. She is always reading books and going to workshops on channeling and things of that sort."

We again underscore that of all the people to experience this kind of vision, it's interesting that it would be Jim and his wife—two people who are not accustomed to "supernatural" occurrences, who are not looking for them in any kind of way.

"You know, Jim," Brad says, "in all of my experiences with traditional healers all across the world, I've learned that Spirit— whether you call it God, the creator, angelic presences, or mystery—likes to come into the lives of people who are least apt to be looking for it. Perhaps this is because when we want it too badly, our mind becomes too much of an obstacle for the holy to make itself known. I don't pretend to know what the green light was, but considering the context in which it occurred, and the fact that it didn't feel scary, I can say that it was a special and wonderful thing you and your wife witnessed." Jim is quiet as he contemplates this information.

"Has your wife ever painted the green light?" Hillary asks.

"No, no" Jim chuckles.

"Jim, if you could think of one word to describe your life right now, what would it be?" Brad interjects.

"Well, the first word that popped into my head was, 'alone'. But I don't like that word, that's not a good word. I'd like to think of another one."

"Okay, Jim, before we see you again this afternoon, I'd like you to think of a special word that speaks to your life right now. Can you do that?"

"Yes."

***

Jim comes back that afternoon and says he called his wife to ask her to help him come up with a word.

"I told her that I thought of 'alone', but that I didn't like it. Then I was describing all my feelings, and she said, 'Well, *alone*. That's what you are describing'," Jim laughs. "But after we hung up I kept trying to think of another one, because I didn't like that word. So I decided on *connection*." Jim goes on to talk about how it's been interesting for him to think about the green light experience again. He shares with us that after our last session he remembered that when he was having a surgery as a child, as he was coming out of anesthetic he had a very brief but clear vision of a sun chasing the moon across the sky.

"Have there been other similar, mysterious experiences in your family?" Hillary asks. Jim thinks for a while.

"Well, now that you mention it, when my father died, that was strange. My father had been very ill when I was a child. He had MS and was blind and could barely move, but he could hear. He was confined to the bed. We took turns taking care of him. I took care of him every day after school. We were very poor. He died when I was 11, at 4 o'clock in the morning. That morning, just before 4 a.m., my mother heard the doorbell ring. She got up to answer it, but there was no one there. She went back to bed, and then she heard it ring again. Again, no one was there. Also, that same morning, my sister and I both had strange dreams and had woken up early, so we were awake when the doorbell rang. That was when we found out my father had died." We express that this seems an amazing occurrence.

"Actually, there is more," Jim said, "Apparently the priest who had been my father's pastor when he was younger—he lived in a different city—heard someone at the bottom of his stairway calling his name, right at the time my father died. He went to look and no one was there. Also, one of my aunts who lived across town had a dream the night before that my father had died. She called us that morning. We found all of this out when everyone came to the house for the funeral."

"Wow! That's a lot of mysterious occurrences in one family. You all must have been amazed to hear that all of that happened," Brad said.

"I guess, but we never really talked about it too much," Jim said. Hillary playfully teased him that naturally this was the case, considering the way they never talked about the green light either. Jim went on to share a few other mysterious stories he had heard about his grandparents and great grandparents. He then shared a dream he had recently had of his father.

"I don't know what you make of this," Jim said, "but I had a dream that my father was telling me something very important. I don't remember in the dream what it was, but I remember that his eyes were a bright glowing blue. In the dream I was so struck by how blue his eyes were, and he was looking at me so intensely. I thought it was strange because my father's eyes were brown. When I told my mother about the dream, she said, 'Where did you get that idea that your father's eyes were brown? Your father had very beautiful blue eyes.' I guess because he was mostly blind when I was a child, and his eyes were dull, that I couldn't tell his eyes were blue."

We celebrate this dream and the way mystery has touched Jim's life and the life of his family. Jim expresses how curious it is the way the memories of these stories have been rushing back to him since he began the sessions.

"Jim, tonight we'd like you to do something. Can you call Beatrice in New Mexico and ask her if she would be willing to paint the green light that she saw that night?"

"Sure."

"Now, at the same time that Beatrice is painting the green light, we'd like you to do something else. We'd like you to take your paintbrush—which by the way, happens to be green—dip it in water, and paint the word *connection* across your chest. Do this at the very same time that Beatrice is doing her painting. Can you do this?"

"Sure, I can do that," Jim says.

"We realize it might sound strange, but it's not important whether or not it makes sense to your rational mind. Just do it." Jim agrees.

***

The next morning Jim returns. He begins by telling us how yesterday evening he went and bought a cigar and enjoyed it as he took a stroll around the streets of the French Quarter. He told us he had been thinking a lot about ancestors and wanted to ask us what we thought about the idea of ancestors.

"Well, Jim," Hillary said, "sounds like you had a very special visit from your father in that dream. Many old cultures say that our ancestors are our connection to God. It is our love and longing for them that keeps that connection strong. All you have to do is think of them and feel them in your heart, and know that they also feel you. The connection is always there."

Jim responds: "I used to smoke cigars with a few of my elder friends who have passed away. Sometimes when I am at home I go out on the porch and smoke a cigar and think of them. It makes me feel close to them." We say it is clear that Jim already knows how to be connected to those who have passed, as well as to the mysteries of spirit. We ask him about his performance of the ritual last night.

"Oh, yes," Jim begins, "well, Beatrice painted the green light. She took a photo of it and I have put it as the wallpaper on my cell phone." He shows us the painting.

"And I painted the word *connection* across my chest. Something strange happened this morning. I was awakened very early in the morning because my laptop in my hotel room all of a sudden turned on, all by itself. The screen lit up just for a second, and then went off again. I thought I must have left it on, and so I looked over at it again and I saw that the green light on the laptop where the power button is. It was glowing and for a moment filled the entire room with a green glow. It was weird. I'm not sure if it was some kind of technical malfunction, though it's never happened before."

"So you had a green light lighting up your room this morning!" Brad smiles.

"I guess so," Jim laughs, "it was strange."

It didn't matter to us whether or not Jim's computer actually malfunctioned or not. "Proving" whether this was a magical occurrence or mere coincidence was not necessary in order to highlight and utilize what had become special and resourceful about the mysterious green light in Jim's life.

"It's very special," Brad repeats, "this event you witnessed with your wife, Beatrice. Now I feel moved to tell you that I once knew a very strong healer in Brazil. I wrote his life story. When people would come to see him he would say a prayer and then wait to internally hear a recipe for a medication that the local pharmacist would make, and then they would be cured. He became very famous for this. His abilities began when he was a small child, when almost every night he would be visited by a glowing green presence. His brothers and sister witnessed it coming to him on several occasions. The boy had the feeling that the green light was teaching him some kind of important lessons, especially how to heal others, but he did not want to do that with his life. One day his older brother became ill and the medical doctors could not help him. This gave him no choice. Remembering that green light, he prayed for help and to his surprise a recipe for making a medicine popped into his mind. He wrote it down and his brother was healed when it was made for him. That's how he became a great traditional healer."

Jim is awestruck by this story.

"The healer never really knew what the green light was, and you may never know what the green light was that visited you and your wife. But clearly, Jim, Spirit is knocking on your door in a good way."

Hillary reminds them that Jim's son was also present when the green light appeared in their family life.

"Have you told your son about this?" Hillary asks.

"No, never." Jim says. We both agree that it feels the time has come for he and his wife to share this story with his son. Jim agrees and remarks that his son is a very wonderful father.

"He is a better father than I was, I think. He has a very kind, calm presence about him. He is very strong, but also loving. Actually, he loves watching those shows on T.V. about ghosts." Jim says his son actually travels across the country visiting places that are supposed to be haunted. We laugh and celebrate the fact that his son, naturally, also has a hidden connection to mystery.

"It's funny," said Jim, "how when I first came here my phone dropped and that sun appeared on the screen."

"And you remembered that you had a vision of the sun chasing away the moon," Hillary says. "A poet might say that the sun is a warm light of connection that can chase away the aloneness of the moonlight." Jim notes that he often feels scared, almost like a child, when he is alone in a dark house at night.

"A green light chases fear out of sight," Brad says playfully.

***

Jim arrives for his final session that afternoon. He is excited to report a recent startling development.

"I just spoke with my wife. Remember, she is staying out with the grandkids right now. Apparently our grandson was up in the middle of the night last night, and he came and asked if he could get in bed with her. This morning she overheard our grandson telling his sister that he had a dream about two green things that looked like blobs, but 'they weren't aliens'. I can't believe it!"

We celebrated the way that Jim, now an elder, after all these years had begun to allow his connection to mystery to blossom into his life and the life of his family. We underscored that Jim and his wife now had a very special story to share with his son and grandchildren, a story about the way we are never alone and always connected to the presence of loving mystery that flows through our relationships to those we love, both living and dead. Jim was transformed by a new awareness of himself as a wise grandfather who, instead of hiding the story, would be able to pass on a gift to his children and grandchildren that could awaken their own connection to the greater mysteries that bring healing.

When the heart is open and soft, music and poetry can enter with a resonance that touches us in ways deeper than any standard conversation. Now that Jim's heart was open, we concluded our final session with music. We asked Jim to sit in a chair while Brad improvised on the piano and Hillary improvised song and poetics to the music. The words celebrated all that took place, and Jim wept.

Jim continues to send us postcards reporting how his life has never been the same. He is now living with more mystery and allows his dreams and imagination to move him to participate more fully in all aspects of his everyday life. He has become an elder beacon of light for those who come to him as clients. As a father and grandfather, he is the wisdom keeper of the family mysteries, the reminders that life is more than what anyone can explain. When the light comes on, it is time to step on the stage and live fully.

Interlude

Every once in a while you hear a rumor about an uncommon client who is on a mission to change therapists. She goes from city to city making appointments with one clinician after another. On occasion she has been known to interrupt important clinical meetings, workshops, and conferences. Be on the lookout for her. She begins each session in a different way for each therapist. It might be a question or it might be a declaration, poem, or even the delivery of a single metaphor.

One time she surprised herself and began without saying a word. She simply drew a circle on the palm of a therapist's hand. The therapist, a well-known hypnotist, was so surprised that she immediately went into trance believing she had experienced something more hypnotically profound than a handshake induction.

In trance, the therapist watched the client dance around her, making a circle in the room. Her client still had not uttered a word. And then she opened her mouth and delivered a whisper. The therapist heard a poem not quite like anything she had heard before. It went something like this:

> In the circle is found a door.
> There you may enter another floor.
> Find it soon and empty the room.
> For in this space, healing takes place.

5. CIRCULAR POETICS: Cybernetic Metalogues and Zen Koans

There is a Zen saying, "Open mouth, already a mistake" (Kwang, 1997). Sometimes this is told to new Zen teachers as a paradoxical teaching or koan when it comes time for them to begin offering talks on the teachings of Buddhism. For Zen teachers who have reached the level of master and carry the title of roshi (literally "old teacher") their "talks" are not really talks but instead called teisho, which translates literally as "'to take in hand and speak out'" (Maezumi Roshi in Yamada, 2004, p. 293). A teisho is not an explanation or discussion about Buddhist teachings, but considered a direct revealing of things-as-they-are, the thusness of each present moment (Roshi Egyoku Nakao, personal communication, May 2009). This is an old Zen way of indicating a distinction between first-order description and second-order embodiment.

The task of giving a talk on Zen Buddhist teachings, which themselves contain the directive that what is essential to teach cannot truly be expressed in words, puts the speaker in one of Bateson's (1972) double binds. Here the problem (e.g., the invitation to say that which cannot be said) cannot be solved inside the same context or understanding in which the problem exists. The teacher cannot effectively say what cannot be said, nor can he avoid opening his mouth to speak. There is no solution. But opening one's mouth anyway plunges the speaker directly into the fertile ground of "no solution," bringing forth another Ouroborean turn in the relationship between the speaker and that which cannot be spoken.

A similar double bind exists for therapists who realize that, despite whatever knowledge or know-how they possess, serving another's healing transformation brings us into contact with unknowable mysteries that can never be wholly spoken, understood, or explained. There is an expectation that creative, transformative experience be brought forth in a context - the field of therapy - that has traditionally inhibited creativity, fostered tidy dualisms, and generally extracted both therapist and client from the greater complexities that hold human experience. It is thus the task of transformative therapists with a healing heart to do more than draw conceptual distinctions between lineal and circular epistemologies or therapy and healing, but to bring forth the radical contextual shifts necessary to breathe that wisdom into being. It is time to "take in hand and speak out" the circular dance of therapeutic interaction. Our profession is in need of a teisho on circular therapeutics.

Transforming the mental health professions requires going past mere descriptions of Western epistemological limitations or the promise of alternatives held by cybernetic epistemology. Instead it requires that our therapeutic encounter itself recursively embody and further bring forth its circular epistemology. We look to the ways in which some of the voices of two traditions, Zen Buddhism and cybernetics, have experimented with the teaching and expression of circular epistemology in ways that exemplify going past the trappings of theory, interpretation, and intellectual analysis alone. Specifically, the metalogues of Gregory Bateson (1972) and the koan records of *The Gateless Gate* (Yamada, 2004) are examined as lessons in the art of embodying the paradox, absurdity, interactivity, and creative complexity that accompanies the expression of circular wisdom.

The discourse of cybernetic epistemologist Gregory Bateson has been described as circular, abstract, obtuse, paradoxical, and difficult, to mention a few metaphors (Harries-Jones, 1995; Montuori, 2005). However, we propose that his form of expression is as important as, if not more important than, the topics he addresses. Likewise, the Zen koan comes from a tradition in which words are used not to impart information, but to bring forth a direct experience of the awakening or the non-dual wisdom upon which the teachings expound (Loori, 2006; Miura & Sasaki, 1965). It could be argued that Bateson (1972) sought to provide an example of his subject matter by the way he discussed it, just as the words of a Zen koan are presented in a way that is meant to embody and enfold one inside its teaching. We propose that this circular, self-reflexive form of expression is more than a literary or expressive style. The teaching is found inside the manner of teaching itself. Similarly, therapy is located in the manner in which it is performed, rather than any of its extracted operations.

Gregory Bateson (1972) proposed a conversational form called a metalogue where a conversation becomes an example of the discussed theme. A metalogue on a dialogue, for example, would be a dialogical dialogue. Its expression would in itself be dialogical. A metalogue on transformation would itself continuously transform throughout its expression. In summary, the key structure of a metalogue performance is the way the topic and discussion about it become intertwined and continuously brought full circle; it is meant to perform circularity. Bateson, a biologist, anthropologist, and transdisciplinarian, was one of the founding members of the originating community of cybernetic scholars. He believed that ideas, descriptions, and communication comprise an ecological fabric for knowing and experience (Charlton, 2008; Harries-Jones, 1995) and his metalogues in particular reflect an effort to express this ecology of mind in written form.

In an even more perplexing manner, the records of koan exchanges in the classic Zen Buddhist text the Gateless Gate (Yamada, 2004) (Mumonkan in Japanese) use language not to evoke intellectual clarity, but to dispel any illusion that any construction of clarity might imply. A koan, whether it is recorded as a statement, poetic verse, or mondo (exchange) is meant to trip over whatever teaching it presents as a way of liberating one from the fixed posturing of linguistic categorization or construed understanding (Goodchild, 1993; Suzuki, 1956). In a way, Zen could be regarded as the opposite complement of cybernetics. Whereas the latter means to organizationally hold the experience of phenomena, Zen aims to liberate any holding. Like Bateson, its means of delivering words are as much the point, not the holding on to any of the words or the implied meanings that can be construed. Here teaching is not paradoxical so much as paradox liberates the hold of any teaching.

We propose that Bateson's (1972) metalogues and the koan encounters of Zen are forms of performance that are less theoretical formulations than aesthetic evocations. Their style is a poetics rather than theory. This is why their expression sometimes confounds readers who try to distill their important points and delineate their arguments. Poetry is expression that refuses to be defined, labeled or pinned down. Poetry spirals on itself. It is inspired and moved to bring forth wisdom, the sacred, emotion, and the heart—central concerns of the exemplary teachers discussed here. Wordsworth (1993/1800) defined poetry as "the spontaneous overflow of powerful feelings..." (p. 151). It dares to discuss the "algorithms of the heart," to quote Bateson's (1972) use of a phrase of Pascal (p. 139). Poetry is evocative and therefore surprises rather than reproduces the predictable. In other words, it is an aesthetic form of creative inquiry rather than a replicated routine.

The poetics of Bateson and the Zen koan are circular. They emphasize, utilize, and embrace the circular interconnections between writer and text, speaker and spoken word, and ultimately teacher and student. Their circularity is recursive in that it feeds on itself, circling back on its own expression in order to generate a dynamic of production and creation of further conversation. We refer to this form of expressive teaching as a circular poetics to emphasize how it is both poetic and devoted to the circularities that poetics allows and encourages by its aesthetic nature.

In the context of therapy, a circularly poetic clinical session is one in which therapeutic interventions and case direction are organized and guided by the recursive interactions between clients and therapists rather than the interpretation and analysis performed by either side of the relationship. This requires a loosening of any attachment to theory, interpretation, analysis, narrative, overly purposeful meaning-making, and other classic approaches to knowing that not only extract the observer from the observed, but overlook the ways in which healing is held inside the improvisational, interactional circling of knower, knowing, and known.

An important caveat: circular poetics is not a therapeutic method or model. You may try to turn it into one, but at some point or another doing so will result in therapy that strays from the second-order circularity that gives rise to circular poetic expression. Circular poetics is a name for the expression of embodied cybernetics in therapeutic or pedagogical encounter (Stephenson & Keeney, 2011). We have given it a name to indicate a distinction teachers of circularity have drawn: bringing forth the higher order circularity of observing/living must itself contain, express, perform, and further invite the circularity it describes. Circular poetics, as embodied cybernetics, is only itself if it continues to re-enter its own existence. Without circular poetics, no circular therapeutics can arise. The Ouroboros must never stop swallowing itself to stay well-fed and alive.

THE CIRCULAR POETICS OF GREGORY BATESON'S METALOGUES

In the introduction to Part One of his famous collection of papers and essays, *Steps to an Ecology of Mind* (1972), Bateson defines a metalogue as follows:

> Definition: A metalogue is a conversation about some problematic subject. This conversation should be such that not only do the participants discuss the problem but the structure of the conversation as a whole is also relevant to the same subject. Only some of the conversations here presented achieve this double format.
> Notably, the history of evolutionary theory is inevitably a metalogue between man and nature, in which the creation and interaction of ideas must necessarily exemplify evolutionary process. (p. 1)

Bateson's metalogues are unique in that they are an attempt to express ideas so that the structure of the explanation recursively embodies and performs the ideas being expressed. But they are also curiously unexpected in their approach, beginning with unusual titles that point to but do not explain in literal terms the topics they discuss: "Why do Things Get in a Muddle?" (p. 3), "Why Do Frenchman?" (p. 9), "About Games and Being Serious" (p. 14), and "Why a Swan?" (p. 33). The exchanges take place between two voices, Father and Daughter, in a tone of conversation less like that of the philosophical and scientific ideas they explore but one between a young girl and her "daddy." An excerpt from "Metalogue: Why Do Frenchman?" (Bateson, 1972, p. 9):

> Father: Anyhow, it is all nonsense. I mean, the notion that language is made of words is all nonsense- and when I said that gestures could not be translated into "mere words", I was talking nonsense, because there is no such thing as "mere words." And all the syntax and grammar and all that stuff is nonsense. It's all based on the idea that "mere" words exist- and there are none.
> Daughter: But, Daddy...
> F: I tell you- we have to start all over again from the beginning and assume that language is first and foremost a system of gestures. Animals after all have only gestures and tones of voice- and words were invented much later. And after that they invented schoolmasters.
> D: Daddy?
> F: Yes.
> D: Would it be a good thing if people gave up words and went back to only using gestures?
> F: Hmm. I don't know... (p. 13)

Bateson's metalogues are obscure, abstract, and even humorous at times, reading like pointers to a larger picture rather than a logical argument. As Harries-Jones (1995) remarks in his analysis of Bateson's expressive form: "Like poetry, a metalogue does not necessarily lead anywhere. It is its own circle" (p. 92). Much of Bateson's other writing, which has been described as "unconsciously poetic" by psychiatrist Rollo May (in Harries-Jones, 1995, p. 94), also embodies his recursive epistemology.

One has the sense when reading Bateson (1972) that we are joining him in his journey of ideas, that we are thinking with him as he writes. Note the way Bateson, in the metalogue "What is an Instinct?", pokes holes in the solidity of even a basic, cherished notion like "gravity" (p. 38):

> Daughter: Daddy, what is an instinct?
> Father: An instinct, my dear, is an explanatory principle.
> D: But what does it explain?
> F: Anything- almost anything at all. Anything you want it to explain.
> D: Don't be silly. It doesn't explain gravity.
> F: No. But that is because nobody wants "instinct" to explain gravity. If they did, it would explain it. We could simply say that the moon has an instinct whose strength varies inversely as the square of the distance...
> D: But that's nonsense, Daddy.
> F: Yes, surely. But it was you who mentioned "instinct," not I.
> D: All right- but then what does explain gravity?
> F: Nothing, my dear, because gravity is an explanatory principle.
> D: Oh. (p. 38)

Having been taught in school that gravity is what makes things fall or stick to the ground, being told that it is an unexplainable explanatory principle is like driving a conceptual wedge in the mind through the name and the thing named. Here Bateson (1972) creates a kind of tiny air pocket of infinity in which the space between the moon and the pointing finger is made visible. Studying Bateson means following him into that space, sorting through the orders of difference inside difference itself without ever retreating back into the stable ground of material "thingishness."

In part the genius of Bateson's writing is the way he seems intent, despite the limits of language, on keeping our knowing suspended inside this conceptual hair's breadth of space in which his "news of a difference'" is found to dance (Bateson, 1972, p. 460). Fond of adopting Jung's distinction between the pleroma (the world of no distinctions, that which is neither full nor empty) and creatura (the world of form and distinctions) (Bateson, 1972, p. 462), Bateson somehow hints that he is aware that even his own explanations are inseparable from the not one, not-two pleroma/creatura dynamic. He does his best to perform the koan "open mouth, already a mistake."

Bateson spent his life imploring scientists and behavioral scientists to recognize the cybernetic circularity of mind, and attended to what many of the advocates of a relational epistemology in systemic therapy omit: the effective pointing out of the gap between name and thing named that is itself the matrix of connection and interactivity, the domain of enacted circularity. Speaking of Bateson, a former student remembers:

> He taught a lot of bits of information, data from experiments, from experience, from art, from poems and savory quotations he loved to recite, which were in and of themselves not 'it'. They were, rather, illustrative of 'it'. They were, a sort of carrier wave... (Nachmanovitch in Harries-Jones, 1995, p. 99).

It could be said that Bateson's deliberate use of expression as a "carrier wave" reflects his efforts to stay teetering on the knife edge between description and the thing itself, that place where description and thing are not separate and yet never quite meet. The "not one, not two" or "not map, not territory" zone is the nonmaterial communicational (creatura) world where difference resides, interacts, and moves circularly and recursively. Any indication of this groundless terrain cannot be spoken, but only hinted at with an embodied difference that resonates with that which cannot be named. The carrier waves of this resonance reside inside the discourse of circular poetics.

Circular poetics in therapy emerges when we ride like a surfer inside the sweet spot of a carrier wave where whatever is distinguished arises from the whole but does not break or collapse back into it. It is this suspension inside separation/connection or distinction/whole that characterizes the performance of circular poetics. Surfing depends upon the ability to distinguish the ocean from the wave and ride the moment of their co-arising. The place of distinction between ocean and wave where water begins and water ends cannot be pinpointed exactly, and yet it is there and felt inside the bones and body of the surfer. This is what it means to be guided by interactivity. Here knowing is explored inside not-knowing, distinctions are explored inside relationship, and a therapist feels inside his or her bones whether a session has fallen in or out of the groove, a client has become stuck or liberated from an understanding, or if they have both forgotten that "gravity," "problems," "solutions," and "therapy" are all invented.

Sometimes a session comes alive the moment we walk into the room and say something uninteresting like, "What brings you here today?" At other times, it takes stirring in a lot of creative inquiries before a single direction takes hold, carrying the session into more fertile ground. Try too hard to be spontaneous, and it may feel contrived. But try ridiculously too hard to do the obvious, and you might step into the magical trapdoor that moves the interaction into another experiential reality. There is no right way; only many possible moves.

Bateson's successful metalogues, like effective therapy, move between and across different forms of expression, including both old and new questions and recommendations, always keeping the circularity of the expected and the unexpected in a stir. Do something different in a session. If that doesn't work, change anything. Change again. Then do more of the same for a moment if it seems to make a difference. Trust your instinct. In the circular poetics of therapeutic encounter you are free to use "instinct" to explain the gravity of any situation, without knowing anything at all about "instinct." Or better yet, trust your instinct and listen to your gut, all the while following your heart.

THE CIRCULAR POETICS OF THE ZEN KOAN

Zen master Isshu Miura (Miura & Fuller Sasaki, 1965) writes that "Zen is 'without words, without explanations, without instruction, without knowledge'. Zen is self-awakening only. Yet if we want to communicate something about it to others, we are forced to fall back on words" (p. 35). One form Zen Buddhist teaching takes through words is the koan, which is loosely translated as a posted, public question or exchange. Maezumi Roshi (in Yamada, 2004), founder of the Zen Center of Los Angeles indicates that a koan

> is much more than a paradoxical riddle designed to prod the mind into intuitive insight. The koan is quite literally a touchstone of reality. It records an instance in which a key issue of practice and realization is presented and examined by experience rather than by

discursive or lineal logic. (p. 293)

The literary history of koans is disputed, but they are said to have originated in China and come into practice in the Japanese Zen tradition by Rinzai master Nan-yuan Hui-yung (Dumoulin, 2006/1988). There are two primary collections of Zen Buddhist koans: *The Gateless Gate* (*Mumonkan* in Japanese) and *The Blue Cliff Record*. There are many translated versions of these, and they include not only the koans themselves, called "cases," but also a Zen master's commentary or teisho on the case. Below we mostly use examples drawn from Koun Yamada Roshi's (2004) translation of the *Mumonkan* or *The Gateless Gate,* a collection of koans compiled in the 13th Century by Chinese Zen master Wumen Hu-k'ai (Mumon Ekai in Japanese). This collection includes commentary by Mumon himself, as well as teisho on the cases by Yamada Roshi.

Like all forms of Buddhist practice and teaching, the koan is above all else a tool for bringing forth a direct experience of what in Buddhism is called enlightenment or awakening (Loori, 2006). Using a cybernetic metaphor, one could say that awakening is the continuous recursive entrance into higher order being. It is not a static state of mind, "higher stage of consciousness," or the adoption of a new philosophy. The moment "awakening" is frozen like this in description it ceases to be awakening. This is in part why Zen koans, in both their written form and in their utilization in transformative interaction, perhaps most exemplify a circular poetic dance between pointing to awakening and awakening itself.

Goodchild (1993) points out that koans skillfully use words to point to that which is not ultimately located in description:

> While it is impossible to define and conceptualize the fundamental insights of Buddhism, it is possible to construct problems, senses, paradoxes, and repeated differences which function as triggers so that such fundamental insights can occur. Then, instead of attempting to incarnate such insights as the expressed content of language, to which they are fundamentally heterogeneous, we may allow language to point beyond itself towards the source of its meaning. (Conclusion, para. 3)

The Gateless Gate itself contains many cases that deal with the problem of getting caught in descriptions. Therapists may regard Zen Buddhist teachings as the antithesis of interpretive psychotherapy in that the teachings balk at even the slightest construction or attachment to interpretation or narrative (Suzuki & Barrett, 1956; Suzuki & Dixon, 2006). In the preface to *The Gateless Gate,* Mumon himself warns against the trap of seeking enlightenment through a collection of words and koans:

> Such remarks are just like raising heavy waves when there is no wind or gouging a wound into fine skin. How much more ridiculous to adhere to words and phrases or try to understand by means of intellect. It is exactly like trying to strike the moon with a stick or to scratch an itchy spot on the foot through the surface of the shoe. What concern do they have with reality? (p. 7).

Fast forward a few hundred years, and a therapist whose heart is on fire with the desire to be a great therapist is wondering how to pass through the gateless gate and help keep a teenage client from dropping out of school. Is it possible to situate the relative smallness of the day to day inside a vast wisdom? Is all therapy a futile attempt to strike the moon with a stick? Can a therapist become a Zen master? And if so can he or she remain a therapist?

Such questions may well best be asked and answered in the form of Zen mondo. Mondo means literally "question and answer" (Suzuki, 1970, p. 28), and describes the various recorded exchanges between students and masters over generations (many of which are recorded as koan cases). But Zen mondo is not a discursive, intellectual dialogue about spiritual matters. Rather it is an exchange that uses words to point beyond words to what in Zen might be called the direct experience of experience. Mondo is the interruption of the logic of the thinking mind, which in Zen is viewed as a barrier to a more complex, whole, experiential knowing (Suzuki, 1970).

In his discussion of Zen mondo, D.T. Suzuki (1970) notes that when a question is posed in dialogic language, naturally there is the potential for intellectualization to arise. If this is nurtured in the exchange, Zen becomes nothing more than mere philosophy: "When a mondo comes to this pass, there must be a turning point which puts an end to the whole procedure" (p. 36). In other words, when a student of therapy asks the professor whether it is social or individual characteristics that shape a person's way of being, the professor may hand the student an apple and ask her if it tastes like the letter "A". But only, of course, if the teacher wants to initiate a context inside which the relationship to knowledge and understanding can be turned and transformed in interesting ways. Likewise, if a therapy session feels stuck or lost inside an endless back-and-forth explanation about a problem, it is time to put an end to that procedure by going outside the box of expected communication.

Mondo attempts to contain the question, the questioner, the responder, the response, and all levels of absolute and relative realities in between. Suzuki (1970) describes a mondo between Sung dynasty monk Chosui Shiye and master Roya Hyoryo. Chosui asks,

> The Originally Pure—how can the mountains and the rivers and the great earth come out of it? The master answered, "The Originally Pure—how can the mountains and the rivers and the great earth come out of it?" (p. 29).

Suzuki then offers this rather circular poetic commentary:

> The answer and the question come out of the same root. Therefore, when the root of the question is taken hold of, the answer is already in our hands without our being conscious of that fact... God by creating a world answers his own question. Chosui understood his question when he saw it echoed back in the form of his own question. This echoing is the answer... The knocking at the door is answered by its being opened. In fact, the knocking is the opening. John calls out to Harry, and Harry responds. The calling is the responding. When this is understood, there is Zen. (p. 30)

Now of course it would be ridiculous to concretize this particular mondo and begin answering all clients' questions by repeating their questions back to them. This misses the point of mondo, which is to cut through conceptual thinking and enter into the improvisational encounter of thusness, or what has been affectionately called the "Tao of now." What feels wise and true in one moment can feel stupid and off the next. If a session screams for the miracle question, then ask it. But don't turn that mondo into a model. Instead be available to be guided by the unknown. The next session may ask for a "catastrophe question." Or a "whatever question." If these questions wake up the sessions, please do not create catastrophe-focused therapy or whatever-focused therapy and apply those models to every client you see, robbing you of the opportunity for your interactions to invent new questions.

Zen mondo and koans are recorded moments of circular poetics that contain a pointing to the ways in which circular expression may come forth anew inside each session. Reading them can inspire a distinction between interpretive dialogue and a dialogic dance of crazy wisdom, but repeating them or trying to reproduce their flavor pulls one out of the circle of dynamic interaction in which the openings for creative transformation are found.

This is in part the teaching of Case 39, "Unmon and a Mistake in Speech":

> THE CASE
> A monk once asked Unmon, "The radiance serenely illuminates the whole vast universe..." Before he could finish the first line, Unmon suddenly interrupted, "Aren't those the words of Chosetsu Shusai?" The monk replied, "Yes, they are." Unmon said, "You have slipped up in the words."
>
> Afterwards, Zen Master Shishin brought the matter up and said, "Tell me, at what point did he slip?"
>
> THE VERSE
> Angling in a swift stream,
> Those greedy for bait will be caught;
> If you open your mouth even a bit,
> Your life will be lost. (p. 185).

We find in Mumon's commentary on the case (pp. 186-7) that this exchange is also a teaching on rote therapy. According to Mumon, Unmon was scolding the monk for repeating the words of Chosetu's verse, written after

Chosetsu's own enlightenment experience:

> When he quoted from Chosetsu's verse, "The radiance serenely illuminates the whole vast universe..." the monk was thinking of these words as Chosetsu's poem. He was, so to speak, looking for the radiance outside of himself. Without a moment's delay, Unmon gave a thrust saying, "Aren't those the words of Chosetsu Shusai?" which means, "Isn't that a borrowed feather?"... We must all see our own radiance within ourselves. (p. 187)

Much of what passes for therapeutic techniques are the "borrowed feathers" of the therapy field where descriptions of transformative experience are mistaken for transformation itself. In the foreword to *The Gateless Gate* (Habito in Yamada, 2004), a former student of Yamada Roshi writes that his teacher warned of students becoming "sidetracked" from their Zen practice when they have breakthrough experiences of awakening because they want to "idealize that experience, memorialize it, and cling to it" (p. xii). It is a common warning of Zen teachers that we kill any insight the moment we attempt to keep it alive in the fixed world of form.

As therapists we can take this lesson into our sessions and remember that our best discoveries, ideas, concepts, models, and maps risk losing their creative, transformative presence once they become concretized in the past (and the past is always only a moment away). Each piece of wisdom has its place; its expression is true for itself in its own way, in its time, and ought to be shared and utilized in a such a way that invites its meaning to be generative of the creative fabric in which it was birthed. Let us be careful not to extract our discoveries from the continuous movement of creative presence in therapeutic interaction. An alternative is to begin offering them up to be digested and performed like the koan exchanges of ancient times, not memorized and regurgitated like old, worn relics of an idea that is now only a two-dimensional picture of what was.

It is important, however, not to take this suggestion too literally. We are not suggesting that either therapists or teachers of therapy not discuss old ideas, never repeat great tools and exercises, or behave as if yesterday never happened. To do so would also be to ignore the recursive, relational dynamic of living experience and become too conceptually stuck in an effort to be creative in our therapy or non-reproductive in our pedagogy. Just think if the monk had never "slipped up in the words," the gift of that koan exchange would never have occurred. Better to be "greedy for bait" and risk getting caught in an interpretation than not try at all. Just remember to stay inside the circularity of interactivity and it will generously free you again from your meaning making. A therapy session may meander through a wilderness of psychobabble interpretation before it gets pulled into the more resourceful depths of mystery. In the mondo of therapeutic exchanges are found the mistakes, mishaps, and pitfalls that are as much the ingredients of healing as moments of clarity and wisdom. Keep dancing and creatively performing inside the circularities of interactivity, for they will swallow and re-birth changed therapists and clients with each fresh turning.

The wisdom of the Zen koan is not simply its logic-bending, mind-twisting expression of ideas. The emphasis in koan "study" is on the spontaneous performance of the koan to the teacher. One's wrestling with a koan must be embodied, performed, and revealed in order to open any door for transformation. Here "embodied" suggests the way a person seems to disappear and become the koan, the way a great actor seems to disappear into the dramatic moment of a play. Reading koans can be thought-provoking, but the Ouroborean wheel turns through the improvisational exchange between students and teachers, clients and therapists. Circular poetics happens when we step into this classic distinction between talking about koans versus becoming them, talking about cybernetics versus being cybernetic, talking about transformation versus transforming, and talking about a healing heart for therapy versus owning the feeling for the heart of healing.

Even as we write we find ourselves hampered by the limitations of describing these distinctions between narrativity and interactivity, therapy and healing in a book. We fear it sounding like a cliché, the printer's "ready-made sentences" (Bateson, 1972, p. 15), since these distinctions are not really new. Like the monk, we may be borrowing Chosetsu's verse. We can only trust our instinct that the re-drawing of these distinctions is called for in the field of therapy at this time and thus serves whatever is new about now. A commentary on clichés by Zen master Bateson:

> Father: ...We all have lots of ready-made sticks of letters, all sorted out into phrases. But if the printer wants to print something new-say, something in a new language, he will have to break up all that sorting of the letters. In the same way, in order to think new thoughts or to say new things, we have to break up all our ready-made ideas and shuffle the pieces. (p. 16)

Really, what else is creative transformation but the art of shuffling pieces and breaking up ready-made ideas? Otherwise, it is a re-print stamping of the same old verses of enlightenment: a therapy of explanation but not transformation, a borrowed feather.

But Gregory Bateson was of course not a Zen master. The clarity with which he discerned patterns of relationship and orders of difference in communication did not become fully enacted or performed in the context of changing human lives. The latter is the domain of a healer or teacher dedicated to the awakening of a client or student. Though the therapy clinic does not occupy the same context as Zen, it is appropriate to suggest that helping clients change ought to at least be situated along the same continuum as the kind of healing people might seek in a temple, church, prayer meeting, or some other place people go to offer up their burdens to a greater mystery.

The emphasis in many therapies on identifying, battling, and conquering a "problem" may offer clients a temporary feeling of respite, and it may even set some kind of change in motion. But it does not bring people closer to the heart of healing which contains more sustainable, abiding lessons in the art of loving oneself and others through life's ups and downs. So-called problems are resourceful teachings when recognized and handled inside the ecology of living. Just like Zen masters realized they could not dispel dualism through dualistic pedagogy, it is time for therapists to recognize that we cannot bring healing through modalities that deny the complexity and creative circularity inherent in healing transformation.

Case Example:
Singing to a Lonely Chili Pepper

A young therapist named Ana attended a workshop we offered in Mexico City on giving therapy a healing heart. Our workshops entail a combination of teaching creative therapeutic performance techniques, discussion, live casework, and brief sessions conducted with therapists in front of the group. Our work is always improvisational and we allow the structure and content of each day to be guided by the interactivity of the group over the course of the weekend. It is common for the workshop to weave in and out of teaching and healing such that this movement begins to take on a life of its own. Song, music, and even dance often spontaneously come forth. Neither we nor the participants ever know when a moment will arise for a transformative healing exchange.

Ana had been to several of our workshops in the past and she, like many others, told us that she comes mostly just to experience being part of the healing and sense of magic that takes place. She said, "It opens my heart and my therapy in unforeseen ways every time." This day she tells us that she is experiencing a change in her life. While she has always been known by her family and friends to be a "sad, fearful, and kind of depressed person," starting about a month ago she has become extraordinarily happy. She is not sure what brought about this change, but she wants it to last. She experiences herself giving a lot of love to others, but she has a fear that somehow all the love she feels will somehow end up hurting her. She is happy that her heart is open, but she is afraid. Her sister is Buddhist and suggests that Ana start meditating. Ana wants to know what we think of meditation, and if she should start a meditation practice. The following transcription is the conversation that subsequently took place:

> BK: The mind is funny, isn't it? The mind is strange. The things it comes up with. The thoughts it produces. I'm not sure whether to tell you what I think you should do or not, because I'm not sure you would

do it. I promise it won't hurt, but if you promise to do it, I'll tell you.

A: Yes, I promise! *(Brad and Ana shake hands)*

BK: I think you must do something that no human being has ever done. You must arrange, as soon as possible, to go to the grocery store. You must look very carefully at all the chili peppers, and choose the one that looks the loneliest. Notice which pepper looks most out of place, the one that is most different from all the others. I don't care if it takes you two minutes or two hours. Then you must buy that one. Take it to wherever there is a mariachi band. Sit as close to the band as you can. Take your chili pepper and do a special meditation. Rub that chili, giving it all the love you can as you listen to the music. Allow the music to take all your attention so your mind doesn't think of anything as you gently give your love to the chili. Do this time and time again. Do it for at least a month, or maybe for the rest of your life. Now you will meditate in a way that no one has ever meditated before. Do you like mariachi?

A: Yes, a lot! I love it!

BK: I like chilies *(laughter)*. Wouldn't that be something, if somehow, that chili became your teacher? Or more precisely that the way you interact with that chili teaches you something important. Wouldn't it be interesting, that as you learn and grow in the meditation that involves pouring love into a chili to the sound of mariachi, that one day you suggest to a client that they do the same? Wouldn't it be something that whatever it was that inspired you to share these things about your life inspired me to say this to you only to prepare you for some client? The client is right now preparing himself or herself for you? These things are much bigger than we can know. I don't know if this meditation is for you, or if it is for a future client, or your sister, or your parents, or everyone in this room, or for the mariachis *(laughter)*. It's a big mystery. Maybe it's for a dream that you have not yet had. Or for a special memory inside of you that has yet to be born. I don't know. How much of it you will know, I don't know. Whether it's important for you to know, I don't know. But I do know that there is much to be learned from loving a lonely chili.

As you do so, a light will shine from your eyes that someone in that band will see. It will change at least one note in how he plays. And at least one person listening will hear something they never would have heard before. That, in turn, might inspire him to go home that night and sing a song to his child in a way he never would have before. And that child, because he heard that song, inspired by that note, inspired by your eyes, that child might grow up to write a book. He grows up and writes a short story because he had a dream. He had a dream about a young woman who told a story about her life, and a crazy man who told her to go to the store to buy a chili and meditate with a mariachi band.

Therapy is a performing art. In art is found the heart of healing. In the heart of healing is found a theatre of circularity, a cybernetic zendo of creative transformation. On that stage a mariachi band sings to a chili pepper so stories may set a fire in the hearts of therapists wanting to heal those who have lost their way inside their lonely suffering. In the circle of performance, life is reborn, as are therapists, healers, clients, mariachi musicians, poets, and chili peppers. The tear of sadness is not that far removed from the tear of joy. Ask a chili pepper. It has the magic to evoke that wisdom.

INTERLUDE

This time she posed a question: "What is the sound of a healing heart for therapy?"

Before the therapist could think of a response, a bee flew into the room and stung a dictionary. Not knowing how to make any sense of this, the therapist handed her the dictionary and asked her to randomly open it. When she looked at the open page she noticed one word. This word stood out like it was waiting for her. The word burned itself into her deepest consciousness.

At that moment, our journeying woman became a therapist, or a cybernetician, or a Zen roshi—I am not sure which one, perhaps all. She looked at the therapist and with a smile, asked another question, "What is the song of one word singing?"

6. CLINICAL TUNING: A Healing Heart Voices Rhapsodic Expression

We began our journey toward a healing heart for therapy by asking that our habits of interpreting be stilled. Of course it is impossible to stop the mind entirely, for it will continue asking questions and constructing explanations. But we can do our best to harness this inner commotion and give it less importance. As we rein back narrativity, our next mission is to jump inside the turning circles of improvisational interaction. Here we find that each session invents its own therapy, guided by the circular dynamics that utilize whatever arises in the interactional flow.

As instruments of change, therapists must be constantly tuned so that they facilitate the turning of virtuous circles rather than contribute to the ongoing vicious cycles that perpetuate suffering in the lives of their clients. Circular participation helps tune the therapist, enabling therapeutic expression and performance to foster resourceful circularity—the performance of circular therapeutics. Among other things, we are constantly reminded that momentary conclusions about therapy are inconclusive proclamations waiting for a dance partner so they may face the possibility of modification. Even the distinctions we have attempted to draw in this book need to constantly move in the currents of transformative change. The differences between therapy and healing, narrativity and interactivity, and lineal and circular epistemology are thereby offered to the larger dance that furthers creativity, generativity, and resourcefulness in the field.

Circular interaction helps keep change changing, transformation transforming, and therapy therapeutic, guided by a responsivity to the altering flavors of a therapy session, and the drifts and alterations of a particular school of therapy and even an entire profession over weeks, months, years, and decades. As it is improvisational, we can never predict the results of recursive movement. We cannot rely on the mere presence or addition of a description, word, theory, or guiding principle to keep us in tune. It is in the constant turning of the circle, the progression of improvisational life inside interactional circularity, where we become tuned instruments. We, like our clients, are tuned through change.

There is another way in which we are brought in tune or out of tune with the interactional processes of change. This concerns the way we actually deliver our performance in a session. For instance, how do we look at a client when we deliver a line? What is the tone of our voice? Are we expressing enthusiasm or are we deadpan with little sign of emotion? An inaudible whisper delivered with a calm manner tunes the interaction differently than an emotionally charged performance of poetics that sounds as if it will break into a Broadway song at any moment. The latter has an enthusiasm and energy that helps wake up the interaction. This by itself can help jumpstart a process of change.

We need to pay more attention to the details regarding how we express ourselves in a session, that is, the delivery of therapy as a performing art. We can learn to congruently alter the tone of our voice and use our nonverbal expression in the ways that a well-trained actor does. Asking a client to change with an uninspired, rational demeanor is less likely to evoke any action toward change. Perhaps this is one of the deficits of therapies that have an attachment to maintaining a calm, sober delivery. As Abraham Maslow

(1964, p. 84) discovered, this is not a very effective way to invite one to have a transformative change. He found that when we switch to metaphor, poetics, or song—what he called "rhapsodic communication"—there is something about the delivery that helps awaken the movement of change in the very moment it is expressed.

Abraham Maslow's (1964) study of peak experiences found that it is difficult communicating to someone about a transformative experience unless the way you communicate helps evoke it. Rhapsodic speech uses more poetics, figures of speech, emotionally charged tones of voice, and demonstrative facial expression. Here an impassioned presence serves welcoming change. Applied to therapy, a clinician can help mobilize someone to experience an important change by charging one's expression in ways that are celebrative and change-inducing by their very sound and intensity. In this regard, Maslow proposed that rhapsodic expression is an "emotional contagion" that helps set off an isomorphic experience in the other.

The use of rhapsodic expression is familiar to traditional healers. They are well aware that initiating a healing interaction has little to do with contemplating a clever idea or having a sudden insight of understanding, nor does it mean holding a reflection about non-knowing, non-doing, or non-dualism. It also has little to do with mastering the ultimate meta-model or cracking the code of therapy. Being in tune is facilitated when the therapist steps into another domain of expression where the rhapsodic is voiced. Here the ecstatic joy of calling for change helps attract its felt presence.

A therapist with a healing heart draws upon rhapsodic communication, whether it involves extensive play with metaphor, poetics, exaggerated absurdity, or voicing words with a more musical tone. Traditional healers go further and suggest that healing literally requires an ecstatically rendered song. They are not referring to the singing that is anything like a professional concert or campfire sing-a-long. There is something special in the delivery of a healer's song that makes it transformative. What matters is the ecstatic voicing that evokes and celebrates a passionate connection with the ineffable processes of healing, enabling the healer to take on the position of being an impassioned cheerleader for change. Said differently, the healing heart of therapy voices rhapsodic expression to set in motion the emotion that rallies transformative action.

Many traditional healers claim that their singing is the secret ingredient behind healing and regard their songs as a medicine. Here we again emphasize that enthusiastic singing is a rhapsodic form of expression that enacts a calling, marking, and acknowledgment of the desired transformation before it happens. It tunes the healer and the client to expect change and to act in ways that prepare for its arrival. It is the passionate emotion held by rhapsodic expression that helps awaken a healing heart and ready the stage for the performance of transformative action.

We are not suggesting that therapists need to sing in their sessions or exercise their vocal chords at the beginning of the clinical workday. Nor are we saying that you should never use song in a session. It is better that the interactions of any particular clinical moment determine what comes forth. If you are inspired to sing, hum, or speak enthusiastically in a session, then do so. Any form of rhapsodic expression—whether it is poetics, song, or other modes of ecstatic performance—helps tune interaction into being more transformative, as long as it flows sincerely and is naturally inspired. Therapy inspired by a healing heart welcomes all forms of the rhapsodic, allowing it to arise whenever the situation calls for it.

Brad spent several decades working with traditional healers throughout the world. Wherever he went, whether in the rainforests of the Amazon, the outback of Australia, the bush of Africa, or in temples, ashrams, villages, and remote dwelling places, no one ever asked him whether he was a licensed therapist. However, practically every healer he became associated with asked him if he had a song. The first time this happened he was in Paraguay where a group of elder Guarani healers formed a circle and asked him to step inside it. They were dressed in their shamanic regalia that included beads, feathers, rattles, and numerous magical objects. Their purpose was to examine what kind of person Brad was and determine whether he would be allowed to enter their healing fraternity. They simply asked him to sing a song. Brad sang with all his heart, and because it was sincere and not a feigned performance, the elders said to him, "We can see your heart and recognize that you are a healer who has a song."

Old school—rather than commercialized new age—shamanism sends the initiate into one ordeal after another with the aim of purging all assumptions, theories, understandings, and fantasies about healing. It empties him through purging, fasting, and long-term praying. All of this is preparation to receive a transformative song that awakens the heart.

The function of a sacred song in traditional healing is that it both helps silence the narrating mind (in case your mind pretends you forgot: narrating mind is the inner voice that won't stop talking and trying to figure everything out), and it inspires a different way of being in the world. Narrating breeds endless self-reflection, constant judgment, addiction to interpretation, and all stereotyped generalizations cast by a narrator who sits outside of life, observing and categorizing. When this voice is stilled, a healer asks that an unspeakable complex wisdom outside the reach of language inspire and organize the course of action. Here narrated script is sacrificed for entry into the unnamable mystery we cautiously call the *sacred*.

Stepping into this stream of non-narrated living feels like the life force itself is flowing inside of you. It is the raw uninterrupted-by-interpreting-mind flow experience that athletes, artists, mystics, and healers live for. One moment inside it is enough to change your entire way of being. Whether an ordeal is brought on by fasting or wrestling with a paradoxical mind-bending koan, the intent is to still the narration and throw you into the center of spontaneous being.

Sometimes our interpretive minds are brought to a stop when a personal catastrophe unexpectedly arrives. A major illness, loss, or calamity can radically disrupt any production of habitual understanding. In that moment, our inner narrator hits bottom and faces an opportunity to radically stop its efforts to interpret and understand. Whether it comes through catastrophe or a ritualized ordeal, the ancient healing traditions teach that the moment of short-circuiting the inner narrator is when you can choose to passionately ask for a different order of experience, one that goes past the habits of framing and is danced by the non-framed flow of life.

During this transformative moment, a spontaneous surge of rhapsodic expression may arise from the depth of your being. At the lowest ebb of defeat, the surrender of narrating mind can immediately lead to entry into a joyous ecstatic experience. As Bateson (1972) describes this kind of spiritual transformation, it is a shift from a symmetrical relationship with the world to one that is a complementary relationship, a conversion from dualism (mind separate from subject) to interaction (mind immanent in the organization of interaction). This transformation may be accompanied by a passionate melody that stirs inside the heart, a poetic pronouncement, or the emergence of visionary imagination. A surge of spine tingling joy may encourage a dance. In a flash, the deepest despair becomes ecstatic joy, while any sense of being lost disappears inside a newfound feeling of familiarity. This is transformative healing ushered by rhapsodic experience, brought forth when narration stops and gives way to interaction with the ineffable in a way that fosters I-Thou, yin-yang, and recursive embodiment.

Rhapsodic expression mirrors the heightened and amplified emotion associated with the move from ceaseless narrating to ecstatic participation inside a greater circle of interactivity. When a therapist gets a song, poem, dance, or enthusiastic shout, there is no longer a need to either follow or reject any therapy model. Rhapsodic expression awakens the heart, removes whatever theoretical straightjacket holds one back from jumping into the circular therapeutics of interactivity, and floods the heart with ecstasy as systemic union and non-separateness are realized in a nontrivial way.

In summary, a therapist receives a healing heart—embodies circular therapeutics—whenever these three things take place: (1) narrativity is tempered and given the least importance; (2) one jumps inside interactivity, allowing a session to be improvised; and (3) rhapsodic expression awakens a strong heartfelt feeling for healing. You actually don't need all three steps. Any step, if fully achieved, will bring all three to fruition. If you rhapsodically voice circularity in a spirited way, it will free you from chit-chat narration and throw you into the stream of ongoing interactivity. If you stop your narrating, perhaps with the help of a good dose of paradoxical absurdity, you will automatically fall into the stream and celebrate the ecstatic deliverance. And finally, if you decide to perform therapy as jazz and become an unfettered improvisationalist, narrativity will quiet down so you can hear the music.

In 1932, Irving Mills wrote the words to a song the Duke Ellington jazz orchestra would make famous: "Just give that rhythm everything you've got... It's not the music, it's not the melody, there's something else that makes that tune complete... It don't mean a thing if it ain't got that swing." The same can be said for any kind of performance, including the performance that sparks change inside a therapy session. Whether we call it *swing, chi, life force*, or what the Bushman call *n/om,* its presence is the something else that makes therapy complete. It probably needs to be said again: "Like theatre and other transformative arts, if a clinical session feels boring or dead, it probably is." (Keeney, 2009, p. 1). Moving from dead to alive is the art of awakening a session, and learning to do so requires more than a collection of techniques or well-defined theories of change. It even requires going past improvisational interaction, cybernetic embodiment, or circular poetic exchange. It requires rhapsodic expression authentically inspired by strong feeling, the kind that has the swing of jazz, infused with the life force that jumpstarts transformation.

We now invite you to take a sabbatical from the standard therapy workshop, institute, book, manual, or university classroom and take some cues from those who know how to sing the blues. Attend a Broadway show, listen to a mariachi singer belt out a romantic lament, or join in the melancholy chorus of an Appalachian coal miner's ballad. It doesn't matter what kind of song it is as long as it stirs your heart. Heart stirring is inseparable from healing.

In 1938, African American author Zora Neale Hurston (1997) was commissioned by the WPA Federal Writer's Project to write about the lives of African Americans living in Florida. In it she celebrated what marked the difference between glee club gospel music and the "Negro spirituals" (p. 79) sung in the sanctified southern churches. A "jagged harmony" (p. 80) and "a group bent on the expression of feelings and not on sound effects" (p. 80), Hurston noted, is what uniquely marks the latter. Unlike the uniform, practiced songs of a concert performance, the spiritual contains the roots of jazz improvisation:

> Keys change....each singing of the piece is a new creation. The congregation is bound by no rules. No two times singing is alike, so that we must consider the rendition of a song not as a final thing, but as a mood. (Hurston, 1997, p. 89)

It is good for therapists to remember that wherever we find human suffering we find rhythm and song. Long before there was a "talking cure" people gathered to "work the spirit" with rhythm, song, and dance. This happened across cultures in various ways. It is a human quality. But somehow therapy has become more like a canned commercial jingle than a soulful expression. If therapy sounds the same from one session to the next or lacks any spirited expression, consider that the congregations about which Hurston (1997) writes, though often non-literate and without formal education, possessed a wisdom the therapy profession lacks.

As Hurston (1997) warns, no group can be "trained to reproduce [a spiritual]. Its truth dies under training like flowers under hot water." (p. 80). The same can be said for healing. Whatever potential healing, creative life force that exists inside people who enter our current helping professions more often than not dies or goes un-nurtured under clinical training. Handling suffering with a model, understanding, explanation, narrative, or schooled approach chokes our relationship to the lessons in wisdom and creativity that pour from our encounters with life's impossible situations.

Perhaps we should say that therapy needs a song—both literally and metaphorically. It is rhapsodic expression that is required and a song is its most exhilarated form. Whether it rhymes, claps, is slow or fast, comes out in tune or not, or has any words at all, a song full of feeling carries the heart current. It's not the lyrics, melody, or harmony that makes a tune complete, it's the swing—the vibrant soulful rhythm—that comes from giving a song everything you've got. Similarly, a clinical session needs to be enlivened by the soulful heartbeat of an awakened healer, allowing all manner of highs and lows to swing inside a rhythm that enthusiastically embraces them with the song and dance of change.

We know that many therapists entered the profession because they felt something pull on their heart. They felt called or inspired to help others. We now invite you to pay more attention to that pulling and less attention to whatever your mind thinks it knows or doesn't know. The Kalahari Bushman elders teach that the pulling you feel is the ropes and lines of connection across space and time (Keeney, 1999, 2003). More poetically, the ropes are felt and made strong through rhapsodic expression that includes singing the longing we feel for the greater mysteries of life—of which the greatest is love.

Lift yourself to the highest station of therapeutic attunement and awaken the healing heart within you. To do so, you must be more inspired by the swing inside rhapsodic song, poetics, humor, and dance. Better to rap than interpret. Laughter serves health better than insight. Swing your therapeutic lines and get the emotion of change in motion. We are not speaking of trivial entertainment, but nontrivial entrainment with the pulse of change. Rhapsodic expression—whether song, rap, poetry, or rhythm inside a delivered line—helps you feel like you are literally inside a process of change, sometimes to such an extent that it makes your body tremble with joy.

The Guarani Indians (Keeney, 1999) propose that a healer with an awakened heart is able to speak "word souls," or words delivered with the tones and rhythms that make them come alive in a soulful way. When the rhythms grab hold of your soul and the melodies awaken your heart, then and then only can the fleeting lyrics, stories, and narratives and come back home. This gives us what the Bushmen call an "ownership for the feeling to heal" (Keeney, 2010, p. 268). Here therapy expresses its therapeutic heart and is ready to reclaim all its words, now voicing them with soul.

Rhapsodic expression can awaken our heart in the same way that it does for traditional healers and carry us into the interactions that heal. Nothing is more thrilling than being inseparable from the voice of change that is orchestrated by the circularities of interaction rather than conscious will or preconceived plan. Here we are constantly invented and reinvented as instruments of transformation. In these moments we may feel like singing a poem: Love is the glue holding together the starfishes, sea anemones, redwood forests, and therapy sessions.[2] Love proves that things don't mean a thing if they ain't got

---

[2] Adapted from Bateson's (2002) famous quote that his work is a reflection upon "…that *wider knowing* which is the glue holding together the starfishes and sea anemones and redwood forests and human committees." (p. 4)

that swing. Swing frees the holding so that love can keep on flowing.

Inside the circularities of healing interaction there are no models, theories, or routinized techniques. Nor is there a cacophonic mishmash that contains no rhyme or reason. There is a healing groove where a deeper kind of reason and rhyme step in time with the movement of heart-to-heart interaction. The swing inside therapy not only can sing, it can dance, joke around, rap, tap, and serve the merriment of creative play, all done in the compassionate service of helping relieve the suffering of others. When a session is cooking, you and the client are danced by a more encompassing *mysterium tremendum* or *fluxus complexus* that is orchestrating every expression. Here life is brought to a session and therapy becomes a rhapsodic celebration of life's turning circles. Collaborate with the dancing and singing gods rather than a client's deadbeat problem, solution, interpretation, story or any out-of-step hegemonic therapy model. Do so to experience a mystery that is beyond human comprehension.

Case Example: Handling the Family Silver

The following exchange took place in a three-day workshop for therapists. This exchange with Teresa, one of the attendees, took place the day before her birthday. She was anxious for the chance to present what she called her "dilemma" to us because she would be missing the rest of the workshop in order to celebrate with her family. In this exchange, interactivity moves toward the voicing of rhapsodic expression, providing heart-to-heart communication.

> Teresa: I want to present a dilemma.
> BK: Okay.
> T: I have a dilemma. My son is 19 years old. I don't have much of a connection with him. I come from a culture where we value responsibility. My father is a doctor. I'm trying to show him and teach him some discipline, but he says I criticize him a lot. I think the role of the

mother is to teach him discipline and responsibility. Unfortunately, I don't know how to put my heart into this task. I want more of a connection with him. We both get angry at each other all the time.

BK: (*pause*) Why don't you buy him a large fork? (*Brad motions a fork that is around 3 feet high with his hands.*)

T: What do I do with this fork?

BK: I don't know, what do you think?

T: Maybe he will think I will want to stick him with it (*laughter*).

BK: Tell him you have a dilemma. Give him this fork and say, "I'm your mother. I don't know whether to feed you or poke you with it. I have a dilemma. I'm your mother, but for the rest of your life, I won't know whether you are the baby or the devil." That would be interesting. He would not be expecting that. Does he live in the house?

T: Yes.

BK: So you will have to decide where you will keep this fork. You'll have to decide whether you keep it near the oven or next to the nursery.

T: He doesn't want to be a baby. And I don't want him to be a baby.

BK: Of course. This is the dilemma. But you're his mother, so he will always be your baby. At the same time, he is becoming a young man. He will also always be your devil. Maybe the large fork needs two sides—one side white, one side red.

(*Teresa begins to weep. There is a pause.*)

BK: I can see another dilemma. It involves whether you present this to him at a meal or before he goes to sleep.

T: What is the difference? Do I try both?

BK: Only you would know. You are the expert on living with a devil and a baby. It's a time in his life where he is facing a fork in the road. Which way to go? Baby or devil.

T: Will he have to choose?

BK: I don't know.

T: But if I ask him this question, whether I poke you or feed you, he has to choose, doesn't he?

BK: I don't know.

T: Me either.

BK: When he was born, did you get him a little baby spoon?

T: Yes.

B: Do you know where it is? Is it hidden or is it put away?

T: It is put way.

BK: You should bring it out. Tell him, "When you were a baby, we got this little spoon. Now that you are becoming a man, it's time for the family to buy a large fork." Then tell him, "I have a dilemma because sometimes I want to feed you, but I realize you have already outgrown the little spoon. And sometimes you frustrate me. Then I want to poke you with this fork. I know how frustrated you are, too. Because you don't know which turn of the road to take for your life. This fork is a gift. You figure out what to do with the fork. It's your job. My job was to handle the little spoon. Your job is to handle the big fork."

T: Thank you. (*Teresa weeps.*)

BK: It's all in how you handle the silver. The silver inside the cloud, the silver you hold in your hand. The silver is the greatest treasure. The silver that is passed from generation to generation. Do you have any silver from your previous generations in your family?

T: Yes.

BK: How far back does it go?

T: My great grandmother.

BK: Bring it out. Put it next to the baby spoon. When all these things are done, you can tell your son, "This silver goes way back. This silver came when you were born, and now, here is your fork. This family, and this relationship, is all about how we choose to handle the silver."

T: Is this going to have an influence on the anger I have inside my heart so I can talk to him and have a better relationship with my son?

BK: It depends on how you handle the silver. There's a lot of silver in your family history. It goes way back. It moves from generation to generation. Furthermore, it's used for things soft and used for things hard. It has to be polished or it loses its shine. Maybe, before you give that large fork to your son, maybe in a quiet place in a quiet moment, you should hug the fork (*Brad rocks back and forth in the chair as if hugging a large fork. Teresa weeps again. Others in the room begin to weep also.*) And put on some music that your family liked when you were a little girl. Maybe it's a folk song or classical symphony. Then close your eyes and remember that you were once born. Did you get a spoon when you were born?

T: Yes.

BK: And you, like your son, had a little spoon. And you grew up and faced a choice. You've had to handle all the silver. Sometimes it gets put away and we forget to polish it. It looks dark and hopeless, and loses its beauty. So we polish it and it comes back to life. So you hold your fork and remember those things as the music plays. I think you need to dance with the fork. People dance with a broom so you can dance with a fork. Maybe it's a waltz. It doesn't matter. In the silver, you will know that you have everything.

(*Brad begins speaking with song in his voice.*)

Every treasure inside of you is waiting to be polished so it can shine your light in a newfound way. And it wants you to shine his little spoon. And if you know where your spoon is too, shine your spoon. Shine all the silver, polish that silver, dance with the fork. You might even take the fork after you dance with it and hold it. Take a little nap with it. Take it over to that other side of you and say, "I want some light to shine on the other side. I want a dream to illumine my darkness tonight. Please shine on me. Whether I remember or not, I know if I shine the fork, I know if I dance the fork and take it with me to the other side, all the forks and all the spoons and all the silver gonna stand up and dance with all the mothers and all the fathers and all the grandmothers, all the way back. Everybody shinin'! Everybody polished! Everyone standin' tall! Lookin' at you, showin' their shine! Showin' the way, the way to the silver light inside your dark cloud!"

(*Brad pauses and then begins speaking again.*)

It's because we sat next to each other at lunch and I saw you order a steak *(this session took place in the afternoon just after lunch)*. You then put a fork into the meat and you found that the meat wasn't done *(the room laughs because this actually occurred)*. You sent it back to the kitchen so they would cook it some more. Just like you sent your son to get cooked again. And now you got your fork and some well-done meat. Time for you to have your son in another way. Inside, inside, the silver that shines.

T: Thank you. Thank you.

BK: One, two, three. One: Never understand. Only stand under. Two: Jump into the stream, and know you're already in it! Three: Sing and dance the song of your family's long history of polished, shining treasure! The day you do it, write down the date. That day will be your silver day, your silver birthday. Every day for the rest of your life, make sure that on that date, you get out all the silver. And polish it. Shine it. You'll know what to do when the music comes on and sings to you. You'll dance and cross into the darkness of the clouds that cannot be seen and understood. There you'll feel and feed the shining light of mama and papa and grandmamma and grandpapa and all the old ones before you who, once upon a time when you were growing up, also wondered what to do with you.

INTERLUDE

Our client became renowned among therapists, and many wondered whether she was really a client at all. One day she visited a school for the therapeutic performing arts and entered a classroom filled with students and faculty. She arranged to have two seats placed in front of the group and proceeded to have a conversation with herself. She would utter a line as if she were a therapist and then get up and sit in the other chair where she answered as a healer. The event was recorded. This is what transpired:

Therapist: I have many colleagues who want to move past the models and techniques of therapy. They are looking to spirituality as a guide as they attend meditation retreats, host sweat lodges, join drumming circles, and read spiritual texts. Will these activities help therapists find a healing heart?

Healer: Please keep in mind that spirituality is as filled with narrativity and interpretation as psychotherapy. If therapists replace their psychological clichés with spiritual clichés, it offers no significant change. It may be better to avoid chasing after new understandings. It's better to learn to improvise. Of course, if improvisation gives you another metaphor that yields a new understanding of therapy, look out. Jump off of whatever cliff of understanding you are now standing on and watch how life itself will catch you and carry you on an interesting flight. Life, or what you call the circles of improvisational circularity, is a better guide than any concretized protocol that recommends simplistic generalizations for how you should typically act in all situations.

T: Yes but isn't it true that therapy would benefit from becoming more spiritual?

H: That's an interpretation. I think it is better to say that therapy should be sanctified, anointed, blessed, or baptized in the creative life force. Without the latter, all you have is another competition over interpretation and that too easily degenerates spiritual discourse into being another flea market of narratives to pick over. If you have the spirit, you don't need to name or explain it. In fact, too much talk about it might make the spirit disappear.

T: How do I get the spirit? Is it a quality, a higher order phenomenon, a metaphysical principal, a religious mystery? What is it?

H: Wise healers never define anything that is in the realm of the holy. That could be blasphemous for it presumes we know what we are talking about! How can we possibly know enough to define the greater complexities of life? As the Biblical Job found out, and Bateson (1987) enjoyed reminding us, we don't even know "the time when the wild goats of the rock bring forth" (*Job* 39:1). Words that point to the holy are better uttered as a means to evoke a felt relationship with it. The voicing of these words should be in the rhapsodic so as to convey respect and an authentic desire to make connection.

T: Maybe we should do the same with the words of therapy that refer to change, transformation, and growth. A therapist should only say these words in ways that help them come alive for the client.

H: Yes, that's what it means to be a healer. Sing them if you must. Don't sit there like a boring automaton and give lifeless expression about a moment the client hopes will change his or her entire life. At the same time, don't fake anything. The client's unconscious and deeper listening will hear you are not sincere. You, the therapist, must feel the possibility for change in each and every moment. When this is felt, you will find yourself voicing the rhapsodic, doing so with a healing heart.

T: So the therapist must first be changed in order to bring change into the session?

H: That is a nice way of putting it. Although there is more to it than that, you are already reminding me to change. This is why I sing or dance before I talk with someone about the most important matters of change and transformation. I must change myself from being an everyday dullard into being a healer. I must cross the bridge into healing before my work can begin. This is the shaman's true journey, not some daydream that inflates the ego's narrative fantasies. The journey from therapist to healer requires awakening the heart so that it can rise and expand. When this takes place, mind becomes a small part inside the heart. This is when circular therapeutics—the heart of healing—is voiced.

T: Is it correct to say that the mind must be inside the heart rather than having our mind frame our heartfelt feelings?

H: Yes, the heart must rise above the head, and the latter must become a servant to the heart. Otherwise, our mind just narrates about heart, wisdom, freedom, love, liberation, and all the other words that are just words when delivered by a clever mind. These words must become charged metaphors that evoke complexities of relationship and interaction when they are sung by the heart. Let the heart sing.

T: If therapy is an art, what is healing?

H: Healing is the art of therapy, the embodied processes of change that transform lives. Do not contextualize art inside therapy. Otherwise art, whether it be dance, music, or painting, serves the intentionality of a therapy model. It too easily becomes trivial and rarely rises to healing. I prefer seeing therapy inside the frame of art. There is no need to have art domesticated by therapy. Art is healing. The constraints of therapy are more likely to hinder than enhance its potency.

T: Why not place healing inside art?

H: Yes, let's keep therapy inside healing, and both inside art. Should art be inside spirituality? What do you think?

T: No! Spirituality, as you taught me, is too easily corrupted as another interpretive game. We want our work to be spirited, not spiritual. The same is true for religion. We want to avoid the interpretivity of religion and hunt for the transformative religious experiences of the spirit that can inspire us to be part of the circular interactivity of healing.

H: This is very important. Perhaps this is why wise elders rarely talk about their spiritual experiences, because doing so too easily tempts others to concretize them as lessons, explanatory stories, or messages from beyond.

T: The same is true for great writers. Faulkner, Marquez, and Stein do not write in order for their works to be interpreted. Nothing is more irritating to an artist than some social theorist or therapist claiming that the artist's work exemplifies their ideas. If a narrative therapist claims that magical realism holds evidential support for a theory of liberation, an artist may say, "Stop colonizing my prose to serve your interpretations." Let's agree that therapy is an art and say no more. To express itself aesthetically requires a relationship with processual complexity, something vaster than the constraints on viewing and doing that a model demands.

H: To enter this sacred vastness requires that mind be put in its place. The heart must rise and swallow mind, making it a part of heart's more complex ways of being inside relationship and interactivity.

T: Criticism of reductionism and hegemonic theories, whether voiced by feminists, systemic theorists, cyberneticians, or those in the performing arts, has pointed to how we might do more than talk about relationship and context. We must embody it, that is, participate inside the dynamics of relational interaction, which are recursively enfolded. We sit inside an ecology of circularities. Seeing it from an outside narrator's position, however, removes us from being moved by its currents.

H: We must surrender mind to the rising and falling emotions of heart's motion. Here we voice poetics, music, and the rhapsodic, entering the present eternity that needs no past or future.

T: This therapy does not indulge in exploration of the past—whether it is childhood or societal history - as a means of explaining a client's life. Here there is no psychological archeology. There is also no evidence-based therapy because that shifts the relevance of a therapeutic moment to the future, and misses the wholeness of being in the fullness of the present moment.

H: We are asking for wisdom-based therapy, which is the art of healing.

T: Or we could say heart-based healing, which is the art of therapy.

H: Perhaps we are calling for the art of living, which is both therapeutic and healing.

T: And filled with the life force. When there is *n/om*, spirit, life force, or chi, there is no need for calling it anything.

H: No need to interpret it as therapy, healing, or art. Or circular therapeutics. It is alive and life holds all it needs to improvise its performance.

T: When we feel this truth, we will want to sing and dance it. This calls us to plunge more deeply inside the turning wheel of circular interactivity. We fall into life, fall in love with loving life, and fall in order to ascend to the greater truths that can never be spoken. Though words can be filled with musicality and rhythmical soul, enabling an echo of the ineffable to be felt in every interaction of our being.

H: In the greatest vastness of the sacred, there is nothing. Not even an interaction, not an individual, and not a single cell. There is only the infinity of endless possibilities occupied by anything and everything as it is needed to perform the next sound of eternity.

T: This may be a strange time to ask this question, but I feel that this is the right moment. Is it necessary to understand cybernetics?

H: Is it necessary to understand understanding?

T: I am reminded of how Gregory Bateson was allergic to any form of change, whether it was therapy or dentistry. Yes, he often refused to go to the dentist. Though he said it was because the dentist office held popular magazines, which he detested, it was more likely that he didn't want anyone trying to change him. Seriously.

H: Bateson lacked the interactional know-how that Heinz Von Foerster seemed to naturally have. Perhaps it was because Heinz grew up as a performing stage magician in addition to being a scientist. He knew how to interact in order to create an illusion.

T: Professor Von Foerster seemed to know his Piaget, fully aware that the construction of objects in a reality requires a stabilized sensory-motor interaction. As William Powers (1974) concluded, we behave in order to control our perceptions. Our actions maintain a stable reality —we act in order to stay in the same reality, what Heinz von Foerster called the law of cognitive homeostasis. Though we act like others act in order to see what we are expected to see, if we don't act, we won't see anything. Kittens who are not allowed to move after birth grow up blind. Therapists who do not change how they act never know there are other ways of seeing.

H: When one reduces therapy—and life—to being dominated by the handling of interpretation and fails to see that the way a performance is enacted is itself a communication about what is spoken and how it should be regarded by others, a blindness to interaction develops. An interactional therapist has an awareness of how people perform their lives, a skill that notices that the drama of who-is-doing-what-to-whom organizes not only a way of expression, but gives rise to spoken metaphors. When we dispose the interacting system and restrict ourselves to interpretation, we throw away the context and its manner of performance. Both stage and actors are dismissed, so that only the scripts remain for examination. Minuchin (1998) made this same critique when he observed that narrative therapists purposefully structure conversations that prevent "observing the way in which family members affect each other in their transactions." (p. 399) In other words, narrative therapists act (set up a form of interaction) that helps keep them blind to interaction. As a result they take no responsibility for how their chosen action makes them see the primacy of interpretation at the cost of interactional blindness. They do not see how their acting brings forth their knowing. In my case, I act so as to not know. Knowing is what I want to get past.

T: At the end of the clinical day, I have to say that I don't find any of the cyberneticians being very useful to the performance of my therapy. They helped me be free of the lineal thinking of therapy models, which essentially involve the same structure: first understand or diagnose and then intervene. But now that I freely improvise, I let go of cybernetics for I don't want to get into the interpreting habits of Bateson, Maturana, Varela, or Von Foerster. Of all these, Von Foerster was most aware of the necessity to release the circular raft that takes one across the stream. He, too once suggested that we stop saying "cybernetics." A good magician knows that it is good to make things disappear every once in a while.

H: So goodbye all interpretations, from cybernetics to therapy models, and from religions to pedagogies. Throw it all away. Then allow any of it to arise spontaneously if an interaction brings it up. But don't hold on to any of it. Let it come and go, rise and fall, becoming part of the circularity that keeps our mind alive and thriving in the inventing of never-ending creation.

T: Before we go have an espresso, please tell me what healing is about. What are we supposed to be doing with a client?

H: We are not there to change anything, though we serve change by being inside emergent interactional processes of change. In other words, we are becoming more whole by surrendering to something bigger than us. It is accurate to say that we are there to heal ourselves as much as the client, or to change and transform as much as anyone else.

T: Carl Whitaker said he was primarily a therapist for his own growth and that the client was second.

H: There is wisdom in that statement, but don't take it too seriously. We are therapists for the same reason that we drink a cup of espresso. We are here talking for the same reason and this is no ordinary reason at all. We are here to experience being alive. It takes a poet and a musician to convey what I really want to say.

T: Healing grabs the heel of the unseen runner who tries to chase life away. When we catch him, we recognize that it is the narrator who is always one step behind or ahead of the experience that is distinct from its encapsulation. Grabbing that heel, bringing the narration to a stop, is healing. Or maybe we should start spelling it "heeling."

H: We are healed/heeled when we forget the past and the future, the inventions of pursuant mind. Outside narration, there is only the present, the eternal now that waits to catch you in its arms so that the world stops and does so by changing every effort you make to explain any of this.

T: Our responsibility when a client comes with suffering is first to not succumb to the temptation to explain it, whether we point to molecules, psychological trauma, or societal oppression. We need to dance with suffering, doing so to the music of change. We should collaborate and cooperate with each communication, including the symptom or problem. In our changing interactions, we enter the stream that holds the dreaming and the meaning to find ourselves feeling more fully alive. There we are tuned, without knowing and without purpose.

H: We are asking for a moment of eternity. When we are fully in it, the cosmos sings and dances. There is nothing we have to do before, during, or after. We know when we have entered the sacred dance of healing for we feel it inside our bodies. There the stars play with our questions and the starfish swim with our answers. Everything makes sense here, even nonsense, for it is the passionate music and rhythm that is now heard, where lyrics are the wings of angels carrying us to the heart of healing, the art of being alive that dances life and death while bringing problems and solutions, suffering and joy inside the circle.

7. Circular Therapeutics: Going to the Crossroads

We again invite you to move from therapist to healer, but this time our request is expressed even more through a traditional healer's voice. As healers, we are going to use discourse in ways that may, at first glance, appear contrary to the forms both academicians and schooled therapists typically use. With a freer use of metaphor inspired by the movement of circular poetics, we aim to evoke interaction with something not yet domesticated by map, model, theory, or understanding. This unnamed presence is partly recognized as the change that changes as we change with it. In other words, we will draw upon circular means of awakening circular participation in the art of fostering circular processes of change—the healing art of circular therapeutics.

Whereas before we prescribed a purging of models and their stock understandings, and encouraged an embrace of improvisational interactivity to prepare the transformative healing ground, now we ask the impossible: let everything go, while at the same time, hold on to everything. Do so while allowing the greater circularities of life to improvise you. Rely more upon illogical, contradictory, and paradoxical advice. Move away from simplistic orientations and allow higher complexity to be more fully present. As you enter into the ways in which the unspeakable arises, be mindful that we are addressing matters outside the easy grasp of language. In the stretching, turning, and whirling of ever-moving circular expression is found the voice of healing, the circular therapeutics of change.

Even the circle is free to unwind as well as to rewind again, in the realization that therapists with a healing heart are not bound to any specified form, including that of circularity. We are free to begin a session hoping to walk the line from a beginning to a middle and an end. We may unashamedly desire a movement from what is impoverished to that which is resourceful, however that is mutually defined. We are not inhibited from imagining any kind of change. How do we get from the here to the there in a clinical session? Perhaps by going round and round in an interaction that spins the forward motion. Thus seen, circularity serves the progression of spun contrarian differences. In the spinning is found the weaving of contexts that hold transformation, so that whatever is present may be released in the motion of the weaver's next weave.

This book has attempted to be a transformative ride, first asking you to let go of holding onto any production of discourse, all the productions of narrating mind. Instead, you were led to a cliff and asked to jump into the interactivity that is the motion that keeps un-modeled action, including words and silence, moving in a never-ending dance. You were asked to be inside a circle that never stops re-entering itself, using cybernetics, metalogue, and even the non-held means of Zen to help keep you aware of the circularities of circularity. As you moved forward, you experienced the deconstruction of everything we asked you to hold even though you had been previously asked to use it to let go of that which had been previously given as a ground on which to stand. Now let it all go so that you are more available to use any of it in any situated transient moment. Do so with anticipation and celebration of the changing of how you participate in change. Now let's speak as healers.

The Kalahari Bushmen most likely created the oldest story in the world. It is the first story of creation. In its performance is held the circularities of cybernetics without the latter's formal knowing. Here is found embodied practical know-how that directs healing to step outside the stasis of narrative. The first healers were changing agents of change, improvisationally moving with an awakened heart. Their story begins with First Creation, or =*Ain*-=*aing*=*ani*. In First Creation everything is constantly changing. The dynamic behind this changing is *n!o'an-ka/'ae*. It assures that nothing ever comes to a stop and is still. In one moment you can be a giraffe and then turn into a zebra or a leopard, eagle, or elephant. This constant shapeshifting also can mix things up at random. You can have the feet of an eland and the head of a lion. Any form can change to any part or whole of another living form. In this territory of ongoing change, every creature communicates with all other living beings. There is no sickness and no one dies. Here the vitality underlying life is found in its changing.

Then one day, language was invented. This gave birth to Second Creation, or *G!xoa*. With the invention of language, everything was named. As soon as a name was received, the named form stopped changing. The zebra was frozen in its zebra shape as were all other creatures, including human beings. This is when sickness and death arrived for the first time. The cost of stopping and stabilizing the world with narratives was suffering and the cessation of eternal life.

Let us pause to consider the dilemma that originally arose for First Creation. Since everything changed in the original realm, it certainly was inevitable for a moment to arrive when the whole of First Creation would change. That is, it had to stop changing—a change of the whole system that perpetuates changing forms. Of course, at the same time, this also means that Second Creation was simply another change within First Creation.

This change of changing was a recursion, a swallowing of the mythological tail of Ouroborous. First Creation—the whole that consisted of changing parts—changed its changing way and things stopped changing. At least this was true for a moment. As long as time is named, things may stop on any count of its moment-to-moment accounting. Before time, there was timeless eternity. The movement of time simply marks another way to distinguish—differentiating this moment from another. As we do so we paradoxically freeze the identity of that which passes through time. The new changing becomes the passing of time. Whereas in eternity, time is stopped while things perpetually change.

The tradeoff is eternity at the cost of constant change, or time at the cost of a perishable standstill. The liberated, atheoretical therapist faces each moment in therapy as an eternity—an eternal here and now—with no beginning, middle or end. There is no outcome in the midst of pure process-oriented experiential work. From a Bushman healer's way of knowing, when we punctuate a stream so as to identify its movement from one moment to another, we risk setting ourselves up to stand in the way of the changing that brings vitality to life, the antidote to suffering.

Traditional Bushman healers have learned how to utilize the slippery paradoxical relations between First and Second Creation. A Bushman healer, or *n/om kxao*, can experientially step into the world of constantly shaping forms that simultaneously hold the appearance of our fixed world. Behind the appearance of a world where things are not constantly changing is the original movement of change. When a Bushman steps into this realization – only accessible when one's heart is fully awakened—the world is perceived as whirling and constantly altering all its forms. Quite literally, a Bushman doctor experiences this ongoing change as a spinning sensation and feels his body start to tremble and shake, a sign that one is inside the changing.

Of course, a doctor cannot step wholly into First Creation or else he might risk becoming a zebra, hummingbird, or hippopotamus. What more accurately takes place is that the doctor places one foot in First Creation and another in Second Creation. This intersection of two worlds, like the twilight that divides day and night, is where transformation, healing, and life-changing experience take place. This is the healing crossroads where a therapist is able to stretch across the boundary that formerly held her back from entering the domain of healing.

Healing requires entry into the realm of changing forms. It is outside the grasp of any model. Therapy, with all its models and muddles, too often falls into being a naming game where names draw distinctions and still the world's changing motion. A therapist must walk away from all that and enter the crossroads, the twilight and intersection of First and Second creation, in order to receive and serve the creative offerings of transformative change.

Please remember that we are talking to you with the metaphorical and rhapsodic voice of a healer. Inside this domain of knowing and being you are able to feel the possibility of changing into anything—quivering, quaking, and shaking as you anticipate a forthcoming change that can radically transform you into an unexpected experience. Outside this domain, you remain a human being clinging to interpretations and understandings that dictate maps for habituated conduct, doing so to maintain homeostasis of an everyday experiential reality.

The movement from therapy to healing asks that your heart awaken and move you to the crossroads where you plant one foot in the light of day and another in the ineffable luminosity of night. There dreams dance with the everyday and imagination teases rigor. This is where healing and therapy become an improvisational interaction, not surrendering to one without a shift into the other. This back and forth crossing between a knowing therapist and not knowing healer includes shifting to a not knowing therapist and a knowing healer. Back and forth across the divide, soaring past the distinction to find yourself circulating in a movement that never stops—here is found the heartbeat, the rhythm, the movement of transformation.

The exact moment of twilight is the infinitesimal midpoint between night and day. At that moment it is neither day nor night, but a possibility for crossing from one to the other. The art of healing requires entering a similar moment in the midpoint of pure nameless process and the stilled world of narrativity where everything is stopped so we can imagine it is known. If we let go of Second Creation, we drift into the dreaming and prelinguistic ways of the creative unconscious. There, anything and everything is free to change into anything and everything. If we cling to Second Creation, there is no life, inspiration, or change. We must enter the twilight that is neither theory nor comprehension-free experience. There, the tension between knowing and not knowing holds us available for transformations that are danced inside the crack between the known and unknown worlds.

Recall how Bateson (1972) referred to Jung's use of the Gnostic terms "pleroma" and "creatura" to refer to the worlds of the unspecifiable (with no distinction) and the specifiable (drawing upon distinction), respectively. The latter is where we indicate distinctions in order to distinguish, that is, create a knowable world. However, we sever holistic wisdom when we assume that knowing and not-knowing are a static duality. The same is true if we assume a duality between any distinctions, including pleroma versus creatura, or First versus Second Creation. The distinguished requires a world absent of distinctions in order to distinguish itself. In other words, the non-distinguished requires distinction in order to be revealed. This paradoxical inclusion that requires separation generates a vibrancy in any stretched contrary where each side is allowed to coexist, while at the same time, the tension between the two is not allowed to relax.

When we invite you to throw away your theories we know this is impossible, but you must try to do it anyway, believing that you can. If you think it is a trick or that it can't be done, then you won't sincerely and authentically throw yourself into the impossible task of emptying your mind of understanding. Understanding this very point is in itself problematic if it gets you off the hook. Therefore, throw away your interpreting, naming, modeling, and theorizing. Even if you can't, do it anyway. Becoming a therapist with a healing heart depends on it.

This koan-like directive aims to stretch the dualism between knowing and unknowing. The more you try to un-know the further you get from unknowing. The same is also true for knowing. If you can successfully stretch this apparent dualism, then you will feel an oscillation. Its back-and-forth motion helps you feel an internal vibration and shaking. This is the entry into the transformative crossroads, the twilight of healing.

If you believe you know, there is no stretch. Similarly, if you believe you don't know, no stretching can take place. You must know and not know, giving equal weight to both. Since you are likely well skilled in thinking/pretending you know, it is the other side that requires more emphasis to get it up to speed with its counterpoint. Stretch your efforts to throw away theories, models, and narratives. Make certain this includes those regarding not-knowing.

You are all the differences, polarities, and dualities of the experiential universe. When they are stretched apart a tension is born. There is nothing wrong with this conflict. This is how the web of relations between the knowable and unknowable is held. In the tension of the stretched differences is found the creative life force. If you do not stretch a dualism, there is little tension. The more it is stretched, the more tension is created and the more likely it will be released, in the same way that pulling back the arrow on the string of a bow makes it more likely for the arrow to fly.

Here is found the secret of traditional healing. Pull back the most important dualisms of life—whether they are life and death, good and evil, or wellness and sickness—and then in the furthest possible stretching, the quaking will start. Pull back an arrow, a slingshot, or a rubber band and feel the tension that will eventually make your arms shake. This is what metaphorically takes place when a traditional Bushman healer trembles. When the dualisms are pulled apart, the body shakes. If you pull back far enough, there will be a momentary flight, like the release of an arrow. This lifts your heart to the heavens. In that moment your creative imagination flies.

After you land, you again pull back the contraries and wait for the tension to shake you until creative flight takes place again. This is the oldest form of human transformation, healing, and spiritual experience. It became lost as texts were created, allowing the almighty word to become more exalted than the transformative experience of stretched differences inherent in dualities, held tension, shaking oscillation, and inevitable release into ecstatic flight. We invite you to pick up the bow and arrow of life and feel the quiver in your body as you pull back the string. Upon its release, enter the flight of ecstatic delight. Do it again and again, never ending. Its cycle of pulling and release into transformative light is the illumined pulse of healing.

While many traditions have tried to get past the bondage of dualisms, they too often get caught trying to fight, conquer, or banish either one side of a cherished distinction or the whole of dualism itself. With that strategy, few ever come close to being freed from the suffering a dualistic mind perpetuates. Traditional healing teaches us to not fight the dualisms, but to use them. We do so by stretching them even further, pulling them so far apart that they start to tremble.

Not only does the dualism shake, but the person holding the shaking dualism also shakes. Both the dualism and its holder become transformed. Is the dualism found in the arrow, bow, string, or archer? Pull all of these indications and their counter-indications and be released from that question. This is the oldest way of escaping the bondage of unanswerable questions. Embrace what life brings to you and stretch it so you both shake and quake. In this shaking is a transformation of differences that can change us and deliver us into the heart of creative living.

If we only reside on one side of the difference inherit in relationship—either separateness or togetherness—we feel no life. If we are stretched and then momentarily propelled from this and all difference, we become part of the becoming that holds all possibilities.

We do not need a practice that harshly separates the positive from the negative. We need circularities holding and circulating the dualisms, contraries, differences, and opposites—not to make them one, but to utilize the tension in their differences. No difference means no tension and no life force. We do not want to integrate anything. We want finer differentiations, more significant opposition, and clearer boundaries that distinguish the "this-ness" and "that-ness" of all things. We do so to enable a relationship to be born of opposite sides, knowing that its embodiment wakes up both sides to be fully alive in relation to one another.

Become more of a contrary, a living contradiction, a sometimes irritating difference that matters so that you can help the universal life force flow. Know that non-differentiated posturing and saccharine framings of the everyday make you dull and lifeless. When necessary, take a prophetic stand and declare something as idiotic or wrong, but don't do this simply to be right. Do it to stretch your contraries. Do not easily marry your opposites. Make them more opposite and then impossibly marry them. Pull a difference apart until both sides are released and made available to be subsequently caught by a circular embrace that hugs both sides of a dualistic form.

Please remember that it is not enough to use the mind to stretch all opposites it perceives. We can only be carried into the twilight of healing on the waves of deep feeling. Whereas the clever mind can draw many fine distinctions, including that between stretching versus clinging to dualisms, it is the boundless depth of your ever-beating poetic heart that calls forth the passionate complexities the mind can only point to. The heart is both the home of and the gateway to First Creation, pulsing with every ever-changing feeling all at once. The heart requires no sorting out of this or that, no distinction between sameness and difference, and no end to the distinctions between sameness and difference. The heart does not even require that the mind distinguish heart from mind, as we are doing here.

It is often said among bona fide healers that no one in his right mind would want to become a mojo doctor, shaman, medicine person, or traditional healer. This is because your life must be stretched into extreme opposites that are sometimes more than you think you can bear. Healers often go through hell—personal calamities of every kind, including health, relational, professional, political, economic, legal, and cultural crises—in order to get stretched, chopped up, and cooked by the gods. This is usually the price. It isn't done as an initiation rite or test. It is done because you have to be stretched as the necessary preparation for a release into the greater truths.

Similarly, it has always disturbed successful and virtuous people when someone supposedly less deserving receives God's mystical grace. The obedient and perseverant monk laments why God has not given him a big mystical experience when he has been so morally good and spiritually obedient. Practice, faith, duty, goodness, and the like, are only part of what is important. What matters most is that we embrace being fully human—fully stretched between all imaginable poles and dualities, sometimes those of heaven and hell.

You can't get to heaven unless you are stretched over hell. In the release, you fly over heaven getting a brief glimpse of the holy ground. Though it may only be a tiny glimpse of heaven, it's enough to keep your spirit lifted for a lifetime—except when you are stretched over hell again. The death and resurrection show of an ecstatic healer requires familiarity with both left and right sides, being stretched over the opposites, and not interfering with the way dualities are played out in your life. Here the crossroads launch ecstatic flights into that which cannot be named.

In your clinical practice a difference is waiting to be stretched. When its tension mounts, a tremor will be felt. Do not stop it. Allow it to bounce, wiggle, rock, and roll. This is the movement of transformation. Even the holy must dance with the profane in order for the stretch to take you past their contradictions. This is where our hearts laugh and weep at the beautiful absurdity of it all.

In the difference between therapist and healer, we find the archery of another moment of release, the brief flight that is at the same time eternal and beyond measure. There we become a healer by giving up whatever ideas and practices of therapy we are attached to maintaining. Now we can appreciate that which we must desperately try to escape, knowing its contribution to helping us move once again in the falling and ascending between therapy and healing, the circular highway to creative transformation.

Enter the polyphonic voice of a poet, healer, therapist, cybernetician, and Zen roshi:

We give rise to polyphonic expression that celebrates the ascension into "second order," experiencing it as the circle that closes upon itself. Enter the paradox that emerges as circularity turns things inside out so that openness is born from closure, which is to suggest that more possibilities for interactivity are made available the more a circle has been recursively turned, perpetuating/maintaining/deepening its own circular closure and thereby enriching its capacity for taking on whatever perturbs, irritates, tickles, and inspires. (The tighter the recursively spun circle, the more elastic-like it becomes, enabling it to handle more compensations in the face of interactional perturbations.) The world now leaps from the difference between map versus territory, or interpretation versus behavior, and finds a stream of recursive emergences. The basic unit of experience—for the poet, therapist, healer, roshi, and scholar—is now the recursive function of an operationally closed system. This same form also defines the organization of a cell, individual, couple, family, conversation, mind, and society. All identities are Eigen-identities, recursions of circularities. In other words, you—and every part of your experience—are a circle. More accurately, you as a circle or a coordinated ecology of circles, are recur-

sively operating so as to maintain stability of closure/autonomy/identity, all done as a participant in the poly-creation of community. At the same time, community creates the autonomous reality of every member, while all the latter generate the operations constituting the social.

The circling, the recursivity of a circling circle, is the movement of inter-activity. There is no longer any need to assume interpretive postures toward experience. The latter is a reflection of an idealized observer facing a mirror, believing it has escaped the bondage of the observed. Fixed narrative is the hegemony and tyranny of words over the circularities of life. Its postmodern fall requires less observed and less said, and more in-formed inside performance.

Experiential reality arises as the consequence of how we perform, beginning with the act of recursively drawing distinctions. You can't simply look at something, including your looking, in order to understand. You must reach out and touch, move, and dance in order to understand. As von Foerster (cited in interview with Clarke, 2009, p. 36) put it, "You have to grasp things in order to grasp them."

When thinking turns upon itself, we face operational circularity, the subject of second-order cybernetics. The same is true when feeling turns upon itself. Our heart recursively moves our heartfelt presence to dance inside the circling recursions we feed back to that which inspires them. Again take notice that there is no solitary radical constructivist, but a coordinated community of autonomous participants bringing each other forth. Cognition is a social affair that includes each thought, feeling, and dream. Together we mutually circulate the world we know. It is not enough to move from the observed to the observer, for then the latter is only another observed. We must move to holding the circularity inherent in self-referential performance, which is the basis for all observing and experiencing and being. Communal realty arises through circularities, better expressed as recursive operations that generate possibilities for multiple identities and worlds for each and every one of us.

Circular therapeutics is the poetics, aesthetics, and ethics of change. The art of awakening a healing heart draws and feeds upon everything a human being can utilize in order to become more human. It does not mean any particular thing. It is not chained to any story, meta-narrative, or the interpretive forms. Nor is it necessarily absent of the productions of hermeneutics and narration. It is all that is human. Nothing less.

Sometimes all of this and more are better said by saying less. What do we need to know about recursion and all its associated verbiage in order to gain a healing heart for therapy? We surrender to this question by offering a single poetic line from Robert Frost: ". . . like a piece of ice on a hot stove the poem must ride on its own melting." In other words, allow therapy to melt. In the melting is found healing.

Case Example:
Staring at 2,000 Degrees of Fire

Brad conducted a consultation with a couple in a university clinic where they had been seeing a therapist for several months. There were multiple issues presented in previous sessions, but Brad was not privy to any background on the couple or their clinical history. The following interaction shows how simply jumping inside circular therapeutics enables all kinds of surprises to come forth. As can be seen, the way inside is sometimes through a stretch—holding what the client brings and stretching it towards absurdity, thereby allowing the newborn tension to shake things up and open alternative possibilities for living. Said differently, allow circularities to emerge that evoke ever-changing recursive possibilities. In other words, encourage therapy to melt into healing.

> Wife: Hi, it's nice to meet you.
> BK: Nice to meet you.
> Husband: All right.
> BK: So are you all cured?
> W: Just by walking in the room.
> BK: Maybe everybody's changing tonight.

W: I was going to bring a book here. We'll have to bring it when I finish. I got it from the library. It's called *Mad in America*. It's the history of psychiatry in the United States.

BK: How weird. That's scary.

W: It's really scary. I would have received electric shock 16 years ago. It would have happened then.

H: Or a lobotomy.

W: Yeah. And the way that they advertised it was that it wasn't a big deal. One of the Kennedy kids was lobotomized. Joe Kennedy didn't even tell the wife or anything. He just went and had it done to their daughter.

H: What was the other book that I got you, the fiction one? Was it called *Isolation Ward*?

W: Those kinds of books are actually uplifting to me because they make me feel a lot better.

BK: Then you found the perfect man because no other man would find anything like that for you.

H: She likes reading about crazy people.

W: Or if the book characters have lots of diseases.

H: Yeah. If there are severe glitches in people's minds or in their bodies, she will like reading about it.

BK: Well that explains everything. That's why you're in therapy, because she just wants to pretend that she's a catastrophe. This is really just a nightclub for you. You probably look forward to coming here.

W: We do. We actually left home an hour early.

BK: I bet if you pretended that you were going to come and get lobotomized, you would have the best session of your life.

W: That would be great.

BK: Totally. You should try that for a week.

H: Yeah.

BK: I think your therapist should help you create the worst symptom and disease ever imagined, make it fiction, and go past all the known categories. Then prepare yourself to come next week and pretend that this is what you have. You would probably have the time of your life. (*Brad turns to the therapist.*) You should double their fee. They're enjoying it too much. (*Brad turns to the wife.*) Perhaps you could write a book on how to enjoy disease.

W: I actually used to write quite a bit.

BK: Really?

W: I was an English major in college until I met him.

BK: Well of course you were. Only a creative person thinks like this.

W: When I turned in my papers to class, the teachers would kill them. Then I decided not to do it anymore.

BK: That really is fascinating. How about your husband? Does he like disease as much as you? Or maybe he just vicariously enjoys you enjoying disease.

W: I never thought that he would, but I think that he is . . .

BK: You're teaching him

W: (*to husband*) Tell them about the podcasts. How you listen to them at work.

BK: What?

H: I'm a welder so I stand in one place for like eight hours a day and just stare at like 2,000 degrees of fire.

BK: Wow! That statement itself was like poetry – you stare at 2,000 degrees of fire. Amazing!

H: Actually, I've got a bachelor's degree in sculpture.

BK: Really!

H: Welding is really mind-dulling work. There's not a whole lot to think about when you're just staring at fire so I needed something to do while I was standing there. I got an MP3 player and listened to the radio for a long time, but then I got tired of listening to the same songs over and over again. Then I started downloading podcasts from NPR and iTunes. I listen to interviews of people and they address different topics.

W: He listened to a discussion of pain.

H: It talked about this woman who went to see a neurologist and he hooked her up to an MRI so she could see her pain. I forgot why or where her pain was from, but she could see the pain in her brain through the MRI. It was like a red fire. When she thought about pain it made it worse and you could see a little flame on the screen.

BK: It's like you welding.

H: I've been downloading different podcasts, especially those about people who are having stuff that's really out there. I listen to it for eight hours a day.

BK: I just had a weird fantasy. Some of those shows have people who have had a near death experience where they see the light.

H: Yes, they've had one on that.

BK: I bet. I just had this fantasy that as you listened to that story, that all of a sudden you made the discovery that God was a welder. When those near death people go down the tunnel, they're seeing God welding. God's job is to weld.

H: Maybe people got the visions wrong. If God is welding, they may have thought they were in the wrong place.

BK: Exactly.

H: Arch welding.

BK: (*to wife*) If you made up a disease to surprise your therapist, what would it be? Maybe it would be a coupled knee disease, where both of your kneecaps keep bumping into each other. Or you find that whenever one of you laughs, the other cries, and you couldn't reverse it. You always initiate the opposite reaction in the other.

W: We kind of do that now. Whenever one of us is in a really good mood, we just can't seem to get on the same wavelength. If I'm in a really good mood, then he's not; or if he's in a really good mood, I'm not. I think that everybody does that. I think that figuring out what the other person is interested in, and then getting educated in that subject helps a relationship. I think that's one of the reasons the podcasts have been so important to our relationship. I know that sounds silly, but when he finds things that interest me, it makes me feel better.

BK: I see. He's your research librarian.

W: Yeah, I don't have to go through all of the bad broadcasts. He just finds the good ones.

BK: When's the last time he sculpted something for you?

W: He used to do that, but it's been a long time since he sculpted.

BK: I bet you miss that.

W: Yeah. I worry that he's not getting to do that. He used to sculpt. The last time he created anything was when I was pregnant. That was almost two and a half years ago. I even used to model for some of the art classes while I was pregnant.

BK: That's exactly what I was going to suggest. That's amazing.

W: I've got the pictures that he drew of me while I was pregnant, and I think those were his last works of art.

BK: And that hasn't happened for several years?

W: You did that piece for me and you put it together in a couple of hours.

H: Yeah, they just had a bunch of pieces of metal lying around so I put them together for her. That was several years ago.

BK: How many people in the room believe that this needs to change this week? Raise your hand. *(All the therapists, observers, and the couple raise their hands.)* That's the end of tonight's session. That's the most important thing you can do in your life right now. Everything else we could talk about would be a waste of time. You need to do this.

H: Ok.

BK: You really need to do it. Do it this time, as if the last two years of waiting prepared you to do it in a way that you've never done before. Those years were an incubation to do it in a special way. It wasn't lost time; it was preparation time. Yes, all the podcasts, all the weird fascination with strange diseases, the pains and fires, and staring at the light, everything has prepared you. Everything that's happened to you in those two years has been preparing you to go deeper inside in a way that you have never known before. It is time to bring out something special. What do you do for him? He sculpted for you. What's been your thing for him? Besides modeling.

W: It's really been very one-sided.

BK: Have you ever written for him, since you're a writer?

W: I haven't. I mean, I don't think so. I've never specifically written anything for him.

BK: Good. That's what you have to do. And you have to believe that for all the years you've been together, it's been a preparation for this. All those years, months, weeks, and days have not been wasted. They've been preparing you to truly write something. You've been incubating something that you're going to write in a way that never could have happened unless you waited all that time to be in this position right now to do it.

W: I feel like I have a lot that I've been incubating.

BK: Good.

W: Yes, for a long time.

BK: This is going to be a new kind of electroconvulsive shock therapy. You are each going to reach in and create something so huge that it's going to shock the two of you into a whole new reality that might end up on a podcast. Are you willing to go all the way this week? Really reach in, pull up something and write for him, and pull up something you sculpt for her. Do you love each other enough to do this? (*They both say yes.*) Awesome! Than get out of here and go do it. We don't want you to be distracted by anything else because this is what's knocking on your door. This is what life is calling you to be right now. Everything else thought about or considered is a waste of time. This is the moment that is ready to hatch what's been incubating. The two of you have been waiting to create for each other in a different way. To create how you give to one another in a deeply profound way. To create and reinvent how you are or can be, should be, will be, forever, this shall be. This really was an extraordinary night. It doesn't feel like a therapy room. It feels like you've created some magic in this room. We all feel it. Okay. We want you to get on with your life as quickly as you can. We're going to be thinking and wondering what it is that you're each going to come up with.

W: All right.

BK: All right. Thanks for coming in.

H: I appreciate you meeting with us. It was very interesting.

BK: Thank you!

This couple brings a teaching to all therapists and mental health workers. You, too, have been incubating all the gifts, resources, and talents that life has planted inside the deep soil of your being. Everything that has happened to you may be recognized as a way of preparing you for your next session. It is time for you to step into the art of working with your heart, doing so to bring healing to your client, your practice, and our profession.

Interlude

In the cases that follow, we present examples of circular therapeutics, as the embodiment of circular poetics as performed in the practice of therapy. Transcribed from actual sessions, the details have been changed to assure anonymity of the clients. As always, the cases themselves are the teaching, showing how circular poetic performance embraces the heart of healing.

We once gave the keynote address to the Second International Congress on Psychology in Puebla, Mexico. We presented poems, songs, and improvised transformative interactions with the audience. Our intention was to provide a performance of circular therapeutics.

The following day we were walking around the zócalo when one of the audience members from the conference enthusiastically came up and offered us some homemade tamales. Rather than talk about how the tamales tasted, she offered us a taste. They were unlike any tamales we had ever eaten before.

That night we dreamed the same dream. The woman who gave us the tamales came to us in our dream and said, "Never say a word when you can offer an actual taste." Then the dream changed and she was in the audience as we were giving our presentation just like we had several days before. She stood up and said these words, "Never say a word when you can offer an actual case."

The very next morning we pledged to forever emphasize teaching through live cases. Wherever we go in the world, we perform live cases and use them to organize what is taught.

If we could, we'd offer you a taste of the tamales that changed the way we teach therapy.

8. The Woman Who Married Jerusalem

Brad Keeney: Please tell me your whole name.

Marisa: I have a terribly long name. It's as long as I am tall: Marisa Rosemary Patricia Martinez Gonzales. How's that? But you can call me Marisa.

BK: I would like for you to tell me something right now that you did not plan to tell me.

M: I hadn't thought about what I would tell you. Honestly, that's the truth.

BK: Is this how you live? Are you always in the moment without a plan? You should be a teacher and teach that to others.

M: I'm always reasoning and planning. But I always come to therapy without any preparation.

BK: Perhaps you should approach your life like you approach your therapy.

M: God, I hadn't thought about it that way.

BK: Maybe you should start treating your everyday life as if it were a therapy session. Are you overprepared in the rest of your life?

M: No, I don't feel I'm too organized in the rest of my life.

BK: So everything happens without a plan?

M: Really, I never think about what is going to happen. I always allow things to happen. Maybe it's wrong, because one should have different schemes and you should be prepared for different outcomes, but I never do it. I analyze things afterwards. After things have happened, I think about it and I make the adjustments.

BK: That's wonderful.

M: You should live because you can't be thinking about what will happen, you can't program if you don't know if tomorrow you'll be here.

BK: So you are happy with your living?

M: I don't know if I'm happy, but I'm worried about how to live.

BK: Is it the analyzing afterwards that is a challenge?

M: Yes, that's true, but because after analyzing, I think I've made a mistake.

BK: If you didn't think about it afterwards, you'd be fine?

M: Maybe.

BK: Why don't you do something besides think? Why don't you write a poem? Why don't you live and then write a poem afterwards?

M: I'm very good at writing.

BK: Live and then write. Then live some more and write some more. But do not think and analyze.

M: I have done that already.

BK: Excellent. How about doing more of it? Whenever you catch yourself thinking, start writing a poem.

M: I haven't exactly written a poem, but I will try. Yes, I do write a lot sometimes and then I delete everything. That must surely be wrong.

BK: Remember that writing is living, and when you really get into your writing, you're really living.

M: That's the way I think. I think it is that way.

BK: There's no problem with your living. The problem is that you're thinking about your living. Stop thinking.

M: It's complicated. I can't imagine myself without thinking. I just can't imagine it.

BK: How long can you go without thinking? One minute?

M: I have never tried to stop it. I mean I always have different thoughts. Even when I'm in the car or I'm fixing something to eat, I'm always thinking.

BK: Why don't we use this time today to see if you can have a little vacation from thinking.

M: Okay, how do I do that? Explain to me how do I do that?

BK: Let's try it for a minute. Okay?

M: Yes. How do you do that?

BK: The second you start to think, I just want you to take your finger and touch your head. The second you think you are starting a thought, just touch your head with that finger. As soon as I see that finger go up, I'll try to distract you to keep you from thinking.

M: I can't imagine how you can do such a thing. Let's see, let's do it, but I don't think I can.

BK: (*Brad points to Marisa's necklace which is a chain holding a lot of rings.*) Why did you decide to wear this ring today? Is the ring more important than what you typically find on a necklace?

M: No, I always wear rings. (*She touches one of them.*) This one is like a small eye. It's Turkish.

BK: Of course it is because your problem is all about an eye. You always have something watching you.

M: It's a Turkish eye.

BK: Your mind likes to watch you. Your thinking likes to watch you. Now I don't think you should touch your head when you think. It's better that you cover that Turkish eye. The next time you think, touch your eye.

M: I always do that. I am always turning that ring around.

BK: That is very interesting. (*Brad points to two other rings.*) Which of these two rings is more important?

M: This one. It was given to me as a present.

BK: Is it from someone special?

M: A trader gave it to me in a nice way and that's why I like it.

BK: All the rings are very important to you?

M: Yes, I always wear rings. I do this all the time. I always have to have a ring near me in order to be able to do anything.

BK: This is the story of your life, isn't it? You try to keep your life moving, but every once in a while you stop and look at your life. The eye looks at you. It's interesting. Do you have very many rings?

M: Many.

BK: Like how many?

M: About 200.

BK: That's incredible. It would be interesting to have a session with all the rings. Please bring all the rings to your next session.

M: I will bring them. They are all fantastic.

BK: When you get up in the morning, do you think about which ring to wear?

M: No.

BK: Do you think about your rings?

M: I don't know…There are a couple of rings which I have decided not to wear any more for a period of time while there are others which I wear automatically.

BK: Are you married to your rings?

M: Oh, yes, I'm married to them.

BK: Very good. So, if there's a fire in your home, you would go get your rings out?

M: Maybe. One day I went into the street with busy traffic because my ring had fallen off. I was not going to lose it, no matter what.

BK: Very interesting.

M: I also have many earrings if you want to see them.

BK: When is the last time you were with someone and you were not wearing a ring?

M: Never. I am complicated. I'm not going to take them off.

BK: I notice how you actually touch them a lot and move them around. This is true for the ones around your neck and the ones on your fingers. It is interesting how you slide some of them off your finger and put them back on. You also scratch that finger like you have an itch.

M: I always do that. Actually, I even do that movement if I don't have my ring on that finger.

BK: Are you dancing with it?

M: Yes, I like to dance, but I don't dance too much.

BK: That is interesting.

M: I buy rings everywhere.

BK: Did you buy a ring when you started having therapy? Do you have a therapy ring?

M: No, I haven't bought any lately. I haven't bought a ring for almost a year.

BK: When did you start therapy?

M: About a month and a half ago.

BK: Maybe that's why you need therapy?

M: Exactly.

BK: Have you ever thought of designing your own rings?

M: No.

BK: Really?

M: No.

BK: You mean someone with 200 rings has not thought of designing her own rings?

M: I haven't thought about designing my own rings.

BK: If you did design yourself a ring, what would it look like?

M: I don't like gold very much so it wouldn't be golden. My ring would be silver and it would have a half-moon and a star.

BK: Half a moon?

M: Yes.

BK: And a star.

M: And maybe a dome that is something like a church, like what is in Jerusalem. Do you know Jerusalem? There is a special mosque in Jerusalem.

BK: You are a spiritual person?

M: Yes.

BK: Are you looking for a guiding star that will lead you to a Holy Land?

M: Yes, to the Holy Land. Perfect.

BK: You now have a guiding star with your therapist.

M: Yes, I like to be with her very much. It's good for me.

BK: She shines a bright light?

M: Yes, she's in my life and I do not believe in coincidences.

BK: What if you woke up in the middle of the night and looked out the window and you saw the star and half-moon that is in Jerusalem?

M: I've seen her on other occasions.

BK: You saw her?

M: Yes, I have seen the image of a half-moon with the star in the sky. Wow! It would be wonderful to actually see it in the sky like it looks in Jerusalem. I would like that.

BK: That would be a magical moment.

M: Yes, I saw it in Jerusalem one night. I saw it in Jerusalem because the mosque is there. But it would be extraordinary to see it in the sky outside my window. I would like seeing it.

BK: It is a fact that you had a moment in Jerusalem where you looked at that mosque and found yourself filled you with tremendous mystery, sacred awe, and deep inspiration. That image should be flooding your life. You should be hunting for that image. Perhaps commission an artist to paint it. Without a doubt you should have a ring designed that incorporates it.

M: I will do it.

BK: Flood your life with that image.

M: Yes!

BK: Have it on a wall, carry it in your purse, and place it around your finger. Maybe that's what your finger is itching for, a ring with that image and design. It's like you're constantly checking to see if that ring has arrived.

M: Yes, that's the way I feel.

BK: Yes, listen to what you said. Do you know a ring designer?

M: Sure, I know just the right person who can do it. Today I was going to wear a charm that has the mosque, but I could not fasten it and I was in a hurry. I just left it there. Today I was going to wear it.

BK: I'm not surprised.

M: Really? I'm impressed because I was going to wear it today.

BK: Because I think you're looking for it, you're wondering where it is but you don't quite reach out and grab hold of it.

M: How do I do that?

BK: Let's just pretend. Let's open our imagination and tell our thinking to go shhhhh. Imagine that your therapist and I said to you, "We'll see you in three days." Then we go to your apartment and have a painter paint the walls with this image and we get a jewelry designer to make a ring for every finger, and earrings, and a necklace of this image. We even have a purse designed with this image. We create many things that will flood your life with what you have been looking for. This would be very interesting.

M: Yes.

BK: Really interesting.

M: Yes, I know.

BK: Now, let me ask this: If you had the ring with this special image, would you still be interested in these other rings?

M: Yes, why not, they are part of me, and my life, and my things.

BK: It's okay. I was wondering whether if you found the right ring, you wouldn't be looking for it all the time.

M: I don't know, but I wouldn't leave my rings. I wouldn't leave them. I would wear that one, but I would continue liking all the other rings.

BK: Now I want to ask about the image involving the mosque with the star and the moon. Which of those three things is the most important? Is it the star, the moon or the mosque?

M: I think that the mosque is because I love Jerusalem, I love that city, so that's why the image is the most important thing for me. Yes, definitely, it's the most important.

BK: Have you told your therapist about Jerusalem?

M: No.

BK: How many people know about how important Jerusalem is to you and how you feel about that image? Who knows?

M: I think that my mother, my sister, and a friend. That's all.

BK: When did this begin? How long have you been in love with Jerusalem?

M: The first time that I went was about 18 years ago. I have always loved Jerusalem. Even before going there, I used to like it. I know all its history. I love it.

BK: Really?

M: I have visited it 39 times.

BK: You're an expert on Jerusalem.

M: Thirty-nine times I have visited Jerusalem.

BK: Wow! You are amazing!

M: Why?

BK: You've been to Jerusalem 39 times and you have 200 rings.

M: If you wish, we can go. I have a trip coming up soon. I own a company of religious tourism named "Faith Tour" (*Tour de la Fe*).

BK: Good! So this is your life.

M: Yes.

BK: Going to Jerusalem.

M: Yes and taking people to Jerusalem. It's exciting. I like it very much.

BK: And loving your rings and your earrings.

M: Yes.

BK: But you are still looking for something.

M: Yes.

BK: Looking for...

M: I'm missing a piece.

BK: Your mosque.

M: Excuse me?

BK: You're looking for your mosque.

M: No, I know where my mosque is.

BK: So what is this missing piece?

M: I don't know.

BK: Interesting. Certainly the fact that two things in your life have such large numbers - 39 trips to Jerusalem and 200 rings - says that in some way they must be connected.

M: Yes, because about 70 percent of my rings have been purchased there.

BK: Really?

M: Yes.

BK: Amazing!

M: I don't have any Mexican rings. All of them are from other places.

BK: Can I tell you what just came to my mind, like an image that surprised me? Is it okay?

M: Well, yes.

BK: Many people marry other people, and sometimes people in spiritual traditions marry a spirit, but I thought maybe you should marry a city. Maybe you should marry Jerusalem. Don't think about it. Imagine it. Imagine being married to Jerusalem. Imagine saying, "I love Jerusalem with all my heart."

M: I love Jerusalem with all my heart, that's true, but with conviction.

BK: And no matter what it does, whether it makes a mistake or whether it gets sick or lost, no matter how long it lives, you will say, "I swear to give my life to Jerusalem." I think you can marry the city.

M: Yes, I'm sure I will marry Jerusalem. It's beautiful.

BK: I think you're engaged to Jerusalem, but you haven't gone to the marriage yet.

M: Some day I will have a house there.

BK: Really?

M: Yes, there are some very expensive apartments, but you can see the Old City every day, and I want to have an apartment there to feed my heart and soul.

BK: If there truly was a ceremony with an official, some music, and a photographer, and you married the city, maybe your wedding ring would be the design that you saw - the mosque and the star and the moon. Maybe that's your ring of the city.

M: Okay, let's go!

BK: I think this story could be on the news all over the world. The headlines and feature story would be: "A woman marries a city."

M: Good. Besides, everybody knows me in Jerusalem.

BK: I want to ask you some important questions, but I don't want you to think before answering. I just want you to respond with the first thing that comes to your mind.

M: Okay.

BK: Is Jerusalem your husband or your wife?

M: My husband.

BK: Good.

M: I really love it.

BK: Because the city can be anything. A city can be...

M: Everything there is...

BK: When you advertise your trips, you can say, "I want to take you to meet my husband."

M: (*Laughing*) I can say that, I have no problem.

BK: I know you don't.

M: No problem.

BK: You are a mosque. The fact that you are so alive with this kind of imagination makes me want to go to Jerusalem.

M: Let's go. I really would love to take everyone there! I will take everyone in the audience there without making any profit. If that's what it takes to take you all, I would really do it. It would be a great satisfaction for me. I would really do that. I would be very happy.

The Woman Who Married Jerusalem

BK: Did Jerusalem make you this way? Did it fill you with this joy and this life, and this imagination?

M: Yes.

BK: Fantastic!

M: It's amazing. Do you know it?

BK: No. You said things happen for a reason. Maybe you came here for us.

M: Yes, to take you all to Jerusalem.

BK: Here we are experiencing this extraordinary woman with vitality, joy, humor, and 200 rings and 39 trips to Jerusalem. Then she invites us to meet her husband.

M: Yes.

BK: You make everyone want to find the same thing you found.

M: That's true.

BK: (*Turning to Marisa's therapist*) I think that perhaps what's been confusing for your client is that she's been living out of wedlock. She been living with Jerusalem, but hasn't gone through the marriage ceremony.

M: Yes! I hadn't thought about it, but it's that way.

BK: As you are happily living each day and night with Jerusalem, you sometimes pause as if to think, "What would people say if they knew I'm living with it, but haven't gotten married? Would people say that I need to get married?"

M: I need to have that ring, the wedding ring, to show that I'm married.

BK: Will you do it?

M: Yes, I can do it. I really love it, I hadn't thought about it that much, but that's the truth. I really love it.

BK: I love it too.

M: It's fantastic, beautiful, extraordinary, marvelous, amazing. Even the water tastes different there.

BK: Water?

M: Yes, even the air is perfume.

BK: You are really in love.

M: Yes.

BK: Yes, it's amazing.

M: I want you to go. No one here can say no now. It's really fantastic. You will thank me.

BK: You could be the client who changed my life.

M: You go to Jerusalem by invitation, because God is inviting.

BK: Let's change chairs. You be the therapist.

M: Okay.

BK: If I go to Jerusalem and I fall in love with Jerusalem too, I want to know more about the ring you chose to marry Jerusalem. I also want to know where in that city you hold the marriage ceremony. At the end of a wedding ceremony you must kiss. I wonder where in Jerusalem you will kiss the city. There must be a spot in Jerusalem where the final vow is taken.

M: The temple's esplanade.

BK: You must kiss something there.

M: The temple's esplanade. You go to the esplanade which is the esplanade of Solomon's Temple where the mosque is now.

BK: Would you kiss the wall?

M: I would kiss the stone in the floor.

BK: Oh.

M: I have done that before.

BK: I'm falling in love with your love for Jerusalem.

M: It's something very natural for me.

BK: Do you see how I'm looking at you differently than when I began? Do you feel that?

M: Yes, I feel different, maybe because I'm talking about Jerusalem. I don't know. I feel touched.

BK: I started talking to you like you were an interesting client and now I'm talking to you like you are a teacher, like you are bringing us a message. Do you see that?

M: Yes, that's good.

BK: You need to find the wedding ring.

M: Yes!

BK: And you need to go to the esplanade and be married to the place you love. Then you have to teach others about love, and what it means to go for a love no matter how crazy or big it is, whether you're in love with a man or a city.

M: Love is most important.

B: Whether you're in love with a city, or whether you're in love with your work, or whether you're in love with God.

M: Exactly. It doesn't matter what. Love is the most important thing.

BK: I feel like I'm in Jerusalem. I feel like I'm in a Jerusalem right now. I feel that your love for Jerusalem is so intimate that you are Jerusalem.

M: No, I'm not that much.

BK: No, I don't mean it in an arrogant way; I mean it in a humble way. Like when you love another so much the two of you are not separate.

M: Yes, that's true.

BK: Hearing you talk about your husband makes me feel like I know your husband.

M: Good. That's my hope when I speak about Jerusalem, that people feel that they are already there.

BK: How interesting that we began our session and for the very first time in my career, I asked a client to say out loud your whole name. Little did I know that like a long dream, you have many names and many rings. Now I think your name needs to be longer. You need to have all those other names, but now you must add Jerusalem.

M: Yes, in Hebrew. I like it.

BK: Yes.

M: I like it.

BK: Mrs. Jerusalem.

M: Yes.

BK: Thank you so much for all that you taught us today.

M: Thank you for giving me a new life.

BK: You were already living with it. I just asked you to go all the way and marry it.

Therapists think too much and can benefit by lifting their finger every time they catch their inner narrator or interpreter interfering with their being in the interactive flow. Perhaps carry an image of an eye, whether on a ring or a playing card. Keep it close by so it can be touched whenever you start to be out of touch with interactivity. It's quite interesting that a ring is a circle, isn't it? It reminds us that we are free to choose any circle to be inside, just as we are free to wear any ring we desire.

Therapists collect and wear schools of therapy like Marisa has many rings. No need to throw away whatever you gathered before. Just put them in their rightful place. Have you ever thought of finding or designing your own therapy ring? Would it be made of gold or silver, or something else? What design would it hold? Would it remind you of a holy place, a sacred song, or an inspiration that changed your heart? Find the ring. Or design it and have it created. Marry the circularity that awakens your heart and brings healing to your therapy and everyday life. Do it to change how you serve change for those who ask for help.

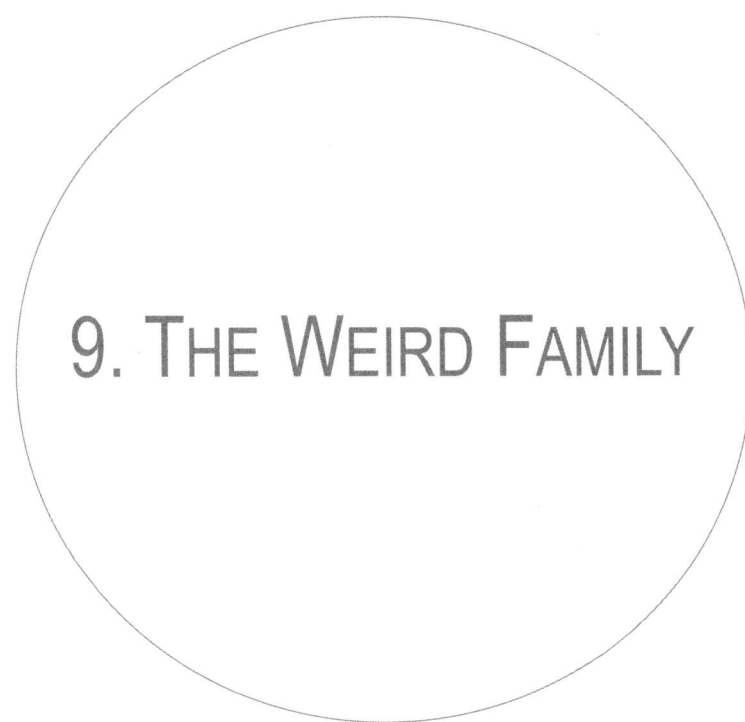

9. THE WEIRD FAMILY

This session was conducted in front of an audience of school counselors from a Louisiana school district. The client was a 32-year-old African American woman who had survived several hurricanes and was living in a FEMA trailer with her two sons. Many of the counselors in the audience had worked with the boys and were frustrated about how to help them stay out of trouble. They disrupted classes and often left school. The following is a transcription of the session.

> Brad Keeney: Nice to meet you, Roberta. Thanks for coming. Why don't you sit right here. We're both very lucky because this is a group of experts watching us.
>
> Roberta: Wow! Thank you every much.
>
> BK: This is a room full of school counselors and therapists who work with mamas and papas whose kids are driving them nuts. I'm sure you want to learn what they have to tell you.
>
> R: Yes!

BK: But what you don't know is that they are dying to know what you can teach them. Because we're all in the same dilemma: kids can be impossible and none of us are sure about what to do when that happens. Are you experiencing impossible kids?

R: Uh, well not at home.

BK: So they're perfect at home?

R: Well, not perfect. They're brothers. . .

BK: One or two? How many kids?

R: Two boys. One is about to be twelve and the other boy is about to turn eleven. I have some "brother bickering" going on at home - little stuff like that. But when they get to school, they just put on something, get into trouble, and people call me 24/7. Then it's a problem. I'm upset because I'm at school too much. I don't know what my boys want from me.

BK: Are they in the same grade?

R: No, my baby boy is in a higher grade than my older boy who requires most of the attention. My baby's getting older. . . It's like they are two different sets of kids. They are fine at home, but always in trouble at school. I just wait to see when they will act crazy.

BK: Can they put on a show at school?

R: Oh yeah.

BK: Both of them? Are both of them entertainers at school? While at home they're a quiet, receptive audience?

R: They are silly while I stay normal. They always tell their teachers that if they are bothered, they will go home. My oldest will take off, running from school.

BK: Who's more talented?

R: My baby.

BK: Is he more talented in getting into trouble?

R: Yes! He's like the class clown.

BK: So I used the right word? We are talking about entertaining at school and having an audience at home. Does he ever watch you entertain at home? Are you an entertainer? Is that where he learned it?

R: No, no, no.
BK: I don't mean getting into trouble. I mean entertaining.
R: Yes, I guess. I love people, I really do.
BK: You could walk into a room and light the room up?
R: Yeah, I mean I like people.
BK: Can you be funny too?
R: Oh, I'm very funny. I'm being honest. I was the same way as him. But I was bored and no one wanted to listen.
BK: Well that's what's wrong with all kids. Kids in trouble are bored and kids not in trouble are bored. The latter just don't have the courage to act and do something about it.
R: Yeah. My babies are really smart. What upsets me is when the school system says they are sorry about all this. I'm the one who is sorry. They're just too smart. What I don't understand is if you give them constant work, it keeps them from getting up and starting some trouble. I had so much work that I didn't have time to act out. When they are grounded and suspended from school, they come home and do work. They sit at the table and I tell them that I want them to get their schoolwork done. I make it just like school. But the school can't get them to work and the teachers tell me that they have other kids to watch over. I understand, but these are my children. I want them to take the time to teach mine as well.
BK: I know that you can't do this, but if you went to school with them, would everything be fine?
R: Oh, I did that.
BK: You did that?
R: When I'm at the school they don't cause any problems.
BK: If you went everyday and stayed all day, would this work?
R: If I had the time.
BK: Let's just say that we got a special grant from the government because your kids are so amazing and they want to try this experiment. If you sat right next to them all day would they would be fine?
R: The school says that before I get there they are totally different.

BK: It seems that the three of you are very close.

R: I'm all they have. I mean we came here after the hurricane and my kids have had a hard life. I shouldn't allow them to be disrespectful, but somebody should want to sit and hear what they have to say. They don't want to get close to anybody else. Because every time they do, they leave.

BK: I think I understand your situation. I'll give you a professional opinion. Your kids love you. And when they're at school they miss you. If you were there and could sit in every one of their classes for the rest of their education, there would be no problem. Right? Then you could all graduate together.

R: I'm trying to graduate on my own. I messed up and didn't finish my education. I've gone back to school.

BK: You are now trying to graduate on your own?

R: Yes, I'm 32. And when I was their age, I was a class clown because I was bored.

BK: Now you are at school together with your boys. You just got your schedule mixed up.

R: Yeah, yeah.

BK: How interesting. Let's now think about some other ways in which you could be in that classroom. Do they carry a picture of you?

R: I try not to give my oldest boy anything to take to school. I'm not going to lie to you 'cause . . .

BK: Do you hear what I'm saying? I mean how can they bring you to the classroom?

R: I don't know. I mean I'm usually there.

BK: I should share my fantasy with you. I don't recommend this, but here is what I was imagining. They could get a tattoo of you, maybe your face. They could then just look at the tattoo and say, "There's mom." If they had a tattoo of you staring at them and then went to the classroom, it might work. Perhaps we can't do that because we might all get in trouble. Maybe there needs to be a reminder that you're with them in spirit. Perhaps they could take your photograph.

(*pause*) Do you guys have a family flag? I know that's a weird thought, but it just popped into my mind.

R: Oh, you mean like a picture on a flag?

BK: I don't know. Here's the deal: the three of you, since you are all funny and you are all alike, and since you're all in school together, and you all belong together, and you don't know what to do when you're separated, everybody then acts out – and you get upset when they get upset. It's obvious what is going on here. You all love each other too much. That's a good thing. I'm serious, but I'm also teasing you.

R: I was wondering. Am I wrong?

BK: No. Everything's right. The problem is how do you get through school with the challenges school presents, when it's more interesting to be with the most fascinating creative teacher they have ever experienced? This teacher is you. Their teachers aren't as good as you are. They don't entertain as well as you do.

R: I'm glad.

BK: Would you say that this is correct?

R: Yes.

BK: Other kids are bored at home. They go to school where the teachers are more interesting. There they find a mentor in a teacher. In your case, your kids found their mentor at home. When they go to school, it's boring and it's not as interesting a classroom as home. I'm just toying with an idea. What can be done to help the three of you be reminded that you're always together in spirit even when you have to take a time out and go to a different place? There were plenty of pirates who had a flag.

R: They know about pirates.

BK: Do they like them?

R: Yes, they love anything to do with pirates.

BK: They love it. They are weird like mom?

R: Yes.

BK: That's good. I'm weird too.

R: I don't understand why they do the things they do at school. When they do really good at home, we always celebrate with a family day. We do something extra like telling ghost stories. Then they'll go to school wanting to share what we did with their friends.

BK: Yes.

R: But when they tell the stories, the teacher gets mad because she doesn't know what is going on. She just sees their friends laughing. This causes problems so I feel bad because when I'm trying to make things good it ends up turning into a bad thing.

BK: It's a good thing when they're doing it at home. They never learned how to be an effective missionary and spread the gospel of your home truth. Right? There's a time and place for that. They have to learn how to set things up, be introduced, get on stage, and all the rest. It's something I trust will sort itself out over time, but I see that it's now driving you nuts and the teachers are lost as well.

R: I never have lied to my kids. A lot of times grown-ups will tell their kids something that isn't true... I have always been honest with my kids and I told them the truth, and that's why I hurt. I'm 32 years old.

BK: When you're with them, do you feel like their mama or their sister?

R: I'm in my house 24/7. I'm always with my kids. What I'm saying is that I try to teach them that what they do has consequences. It's unfair for them to punish me. I'm trying to do what I'm supposed to do at school...

BK: They just want you at school.

R: I know, but I just want to be at my own school, in my own classes.

BK: They just want you there at their school. And it works. They know how to get you in school. When they miss their mama, they know how to get her there. They get into trouble and there you are. Then they're happy.

R: Yes, but I don't understand.

BK: Let's go back to thinking about how you can be there without physically being there. The reason I brought up the flag is because sometimes pirates have a flag, or a team has a flag, or a town or a village has a flag. I'm wondering whether the three of you could sit down together and announce that you need a family flag. I wonder what that flag would be. They will look at you and say, "What do you think, Mom?"

R: I could get some cloth or paper from the neighborhood and have everybody put their favorite things on it.

BK: Cool, like a collage. Just throw different things on it. I love that idea. Does anybody draw in your family?

R: My oldest little boy used to draw.

BK: Perfect. Maybe you should have him draw a design for the flag.

R: Yes!

BK: You all can draw a flag. A flag can be big or it can be small. It would be nice to have a big flag at home, while they could take a small flag to school. I'm not sure how you would do this, but wouldn't it be interesting if they had a real tiny flag that they could attach to the tip of a pencil? When they're sitting in class and get the feeling that they want you there, they could look right at that flag and be reminded that they are still on the same ship. They might think, "We're all in the same ocean. We're all in the same place." I don't know, it's sort of crazy and weird.

R: I like it though. I think I can do it.

BK: There's other things to consider doing. Try to think of other reminders they could have while they're at school that lets them know that you're still with them. Maybe you could write them . . .

R: Like a letter or something?

BK: Maybe a little tiny sentence. What do you call the little one?

R: I call him "baby boy." I call my older boy something else. They call me Mom.

BK: But you're a team? You're a team?

R: Yes, it's always been us three.

BK: Well maybe you should write something like, "Hey team, no matter where we are, we're always together." Just write that and put it inside their belt. Do they wear a belt?

R: Yes.

BK: You could tape it inside their belt, but make sure they don't tell anyone. They will privately know that inside their belt is a message from mom saying, "Hey team, no matter where we are, we're together." There's two things for you to do. First, design a flag—make a big flag at home and maybe a little flag to take with them to school. And second, place a little message from mom inside their belts. If you could flood their mind with reminders that when they go away from the most interesting theatre of their life—the Las Vegas of your home—you are all still together as a team.

R: Yes, is it ever Las Vegas! I mean all the kids who are their friends used to never leave my house. But I love it. You know what I mean.

BK: But they can take all that happiness with them and keep it privately covered up so they know you are all together in spirit. They need reminders.

R: Do you really think that's it? All these years I've been fighting with this. Do you think that's the answer? I hope it is.

BK: I think your situation is hopeless. I also think that this is a great thing. It's hopeless because love is too strong to change. They're always going to love you.

R: Hopeless?

BK: What I mean by that is that the school is always going to be boring. That's a given. We're not going to change the schools. They are going to be boring. On the other hand, a student might get lucky. If you go to elementary school or high school, and you have one good teacher, you're a lucky person. I don't mean that everybody's a bad teacher. I am talking about a teacher who connects with you and you feel like they're making a difference in your life. If that happens once, you are blessed. In the case of your boys, no one can live up to your teaching and your mentoring them. My guess is that you're always going to have the boring thing at school, and you can't change the boring thing. We already know what works. What works is when you're in school with them. The question is how to put you in school in a way that works for everyone. When you're not there physically, how can we flood them with the realization that you are there in spirit? This should be your experiment. I bet that you're the talk of the school and the talk of everyone who knows what's going on with you all, a situation which is like two families. Here's your family at home. And here's your family at school. The family changes as it goes from one to the other. How can we bring some of that home family into the school family, without your life being interrupted in an annoying way? I have an idea though I know you probably can't do this. Wouldn't it be nice if they each had an iPhone so whenever they're ready to act out at school, they could turn on a video clip and there you would be. You could be pointing at them and telling them to sit still and work. Maybe you need a camera.

R: Uh, that's going cause problems. My oldest son . . .

BK: Do you have access to a camera?

R: Yeah.

BK: Then you should take a picture of yourself doing that—pointing at them and telling them to do their schoolwork. Isn't that what you do to them at home?

R: Yes, but . . .

BK: That's right. Put the photo of you inside their notebook. Whenever they open their notebooks, there you are pointing, but be smiling when you do it. Create different poses. Sometimes smile, at other times look serious or be laughing, vary from using one or more fingers to point—as many different poses as you can imagine. Your goal is to flood their minds with your presence. Because when you walk in the room they snap to. I think they are always going to be creative so you must be creative too. It will be interesting for you to be weird with this, because that's what you're an expert in. You are an expert in weirdness. School is a failure because it's boring and not creative and not weird. All the rational things that counselors and teachers try to do are boring. So stop doing that with them. Use what works. What works at home is being funny and being weird.

R: I never thought of that. For real. I always thought I should talk to another psychiatrist or another therapist to see what they would say, but it never works.

BK: No, they're too rational. Stay away from them. They're not weird enough. No, they won't get who you are and how special you are as a loving family with creative weirdness.

R: I think that might work. For real.

BK: Weirdness is what works. It's the mojo this family already uses successfully. It is. . .

R: I haven't said the word "weird" lately. I have weird kids.

BK: Weirdness is just another word for creativity. Weirdness is another word for how to be out of the box. Enjoy it.

R: Well I don't care as long as it works. I'll try anything.

BK: Exactly! I could see you being on Oprah's television network someday. Maybe the three of you will write a book together. Perhaps the title will be: "How to Be a Weird Family"—that is, how to be a weird family and survive school and everything else that is boring.

R: I don't know. . .

BK: Maybe your flag should have the word "weird" on it. Would they use that word?

R: Yeah.

BK: It's a nice word. Maybe it should be on the flag. It should be a weird flag with your favorite things on it, but it should all be weird. And on top is a weird family indicated by the letters, "W. F." (*At this moment a strong gale of wind blows outside, drawing everyone's attention to look out the window.*) What was that? Did you hear that?

R: I know what it is.

BK: I think we're onto something. The wind. Did you hear it? It sort of echoed...

R: Things do happen for a reason.

BK: What are you studying in school?

R: I write poetry and I take pictures.

BK: Really?

The Weird Family 191

R: Yes, my goal is to own my own gallery. And sell my photographs and make a poetry album. But I have to get there.

BK: What you just said took my breath away. I am practically speechless. Because "weird" is really a cover-up word for being creative. The world sees your family as weird, but it's actually creative. They don't know that behind this mama is somebody who's a poet and a photographer who wants a gallery. They don't see that behind your kids at school are kids at home who respect and love their mama and have no problems and are simply bored with their situation. This is making so much sense. I think you're alright. It's the world that is figuring out how it's going to hold you because you're all too creative for the world.

R: I thought I was just weird.

BK: That's the same. You might feel that you can't say how creative you are, because the word "creative" sounds arrogant. So what you say is, "I'm weird." It's a way of being humble.

R: Okay.

BK: Actually, maybe that's your problem. You're too humble. You don't come up and say, "I'm an artist." You say, "I'm weird." Or "I'm crazy." Or whatever makes others think you are not on top of your life.

R: Yes, I'm very weird. And you really noticed, I mean . . .

BK: Yes? Well, I'm glad.

R: Thank you.

BK: What we've been talking about is that kids are often bored, but your kids are more than bored. These are kids who really enjoy expressing themselves and have familiarity with being around a real, live, creative human being who's a little shy and humble about owning it. She sort of puts herself down by saying, "I'm weird." My opinion is that your family needs to take pride in how creative and weird they are and bring that creativity and weirdness to school in a way that teaches them how you can be this way without getting into trouble. It's more satisfying to get away with being creative and weird than getting in trouble for it. It's more satisfying for them to be sitting in class and know that their mind can hold the humor and laughter of Mom. Do they enjoy when you laugh?

R: Yes.

BK: You can see that it's like medicine to them?

R: Yes.

BK: The photographs you choose to put in your sons' notebooks might later show up in your gallery. This should be your first gallery opening. You can highlight the photographs that you give to your boys to remind them that they can be creative in their lives and school. In this way, you'll always be with them as their mentor who reminds them to accept and be proud of their creative talents. These photographs will show you being weird and laughing and staring at them. They should be works of art. Place them inside their notebooks. Do they carry a wallet?

R: Yeah.

BK: Place some inside each wallet. I would even say put a photo inside their shoes. Place them in their shoes so when they walk they're actually walking with you.

R: Yes, they can say, "Mama walking with me all day." How do you feel about that?

BK: I love it. I think that your gallery will some day show these photographs and exhibit the shoes with the photographs that enabled you to walk through all your education and future dreams.

R: Yes!

BK: I think this could make news. Perhaps the *New York Times* will find out about an African American woman who survived Louisiana hurricanes and taught her sons how to walk through life holding their family's creativity by their side.

R: That's good.

BK: Your family's life has been blown around by every imaginable kind of storm, from above and below, but the future can show that you decided that you will tap into your inner creativity, inner wisdom, and deep love for your kids and bring life to the whole family. You can decide to take a stand and be an artist for your kids and teach them that this is the show. What you do with your kids can later go into a gallery where you can teach the world what you learned. That's news. Maybe a gallery in New York will call you. You can become a truly weird mama. Mama Weird, the mother who's a photographer and poet who found a way to be in the system with love and creativity and weirdness. That's a story.

R: You're talking about a lot of stuff that you are not supposed to know about. I was born with a fear. I always dreamed that I could be a lot more than I am. It's hard to believe that you are talking to my deepest secrets.

BK: You are talking about the same thing that your kids go through when they go to school. It's hard to believe they'd be willing to have fun and feel as alive as they are in that situation. They get upset like you get upset when you become frustrated thinking you can't be who you really are. It makes you out of touch with your creative longings. Do you know what? I've seen you here today. I have experienced you firsthand. I know you have an amazing story and I feel the truth of your story. I know that in spite of all the trouble that comes knocking on your door and all the challenges that have come to you and filled you with doubt, you know that you can do it. I know that about you. Because you're strong. You exude strength. That's why when you walk into a party, or when you come to a group of people, they're sitting there waiting for you to arrive because the party doesn't come to life until you arrive. Is that right?

R: Yes.

BK: That's who you are. Just like these boys who don't come to life until you walk into that classroom. You've got to find a way to spread yourself in the world. Not only with your kids, but with the rest of the world. It's not you who has the problem. It's the world. Your photographs need to not only be in textbooks, they need to be in galleries. Someday your photographs should be spread everywhere. Do you hear what I'm saying? I think you are on to something. I think you know exactly what to do. Which is be who you are, invite your kids to be who they are, and then just get some street smarts. Get some weird hope. Not rational hope, but weird hope. Instill them with weird discipline. Not boring discipline, but weird discipline. If they have to get into trouble at school, make it weird trouble—the kind of trouble that's not boring trouble. Weird trouble is a good trouble and you get away with it, without getting into trouble.

R: Okay. I got you.

BK: Good. You're the expert. You are going to have a career crisis because you're not going to know if you want to be just an artist or whether you want to take what you know and help other moms who are stuck in the same kind of situation. That's possible. Will you take a pledge that you are going to follow up with the things we talked about? Are you?

R: Yes!

BK: If you do it and start cultivating some weird hope in yourself, you will believe in yourself in a way that you've never allowed to come forth. You will know that this has happened when you find yourself thinking or saying that you are weird, but this time you will be proud of it. I want you to say "weird" with a capital "W" and not a little "w". I want you to be proud of your weirdness. Not ashamed and not scared of it. If you get that gallery showing, that weirdness is going to help it take off. Because it will be a showing that is unlike anything anyone has ever seen before.

R: I will do it!

BK: The same is true for your kids. You all need to figure out how to change the world through your weirdness, doing so in a way that reminds you that you are always in this family forever.

R: Yes sir, thank you very much, sir.

BK: Can I have a hug?

R: Yes, sir.

BK: Bless you.

R: Thank y'all.

The teaching of this session is that a vicious circle can be spun in reverse, bringing forth a virtuous circle. Getting into trouble all the time is a skill. Not everyone can do it. Rather than opposing the underlying creative processes that create trouble, one can harness them and turn them in another direction. Improvisation in the art of creative transformation requires that we tap into the gifts, strengths, and resources that organize any noticeable outcome and then find a way to help people utilize the same processes to move their lives forward in a more enriched way.

After this session was conducted, many of the school counselors who watched it announced that they were stunned to see what an amazing person Roberta actually is and that her sons could now be seen in a different way. Rather than treat presumed problems and problem-carrying people, we can strictly focus on feeding circular interactions that bring forth the best in people. Here impoverished experience gives way to enriched lives, finding that the same skills give rise to either. Rather than fix people, we can reset their compass and point them to a more resourceful way of utilizing themselves. It's sometimes all a matter of whether the circularities that organize daily life spin one way or another.

10. Seeing a Ghost

When you step into improvisational interactivity that is not short-circuited by pre-packaged interpretations, something magical is more likely to happen in a session. Here we find a client who inspires his therapist to follow a completely irrational direction. The way the client looked when he sat down in a chair, even before he opened his mouth to utter a word, inspired Brad to ask a question he had never asked before, leading to the discovery of a special mystery in the client's life. The client, Carlos, is in his late 50s, and was seen as a demonstration interview at an international therapy conference.

> Carlos: I came to see you because I have a problem related to stress. I get stressed very easily. I am a lawyer and have a law firm. I can do certain things to relax myself, but in a very short while I'm terribly stressed again. I tense up to the point that I feel my joints become numb. I especially feel my hands stiffen up and sometimes my feet as well. I'm worried because stress is affecting the quality of my life. I sleep tensed

and use a plastic guard to avoid breaking my teeth. I'm worried because I am afraid it might develop into arteriosclerosis. During the weekends I try to go to a house on the outskirts of town to have a massage and take a hot bath. I have a doctor who provides me with relaxation therapy, but though I have improved quite a lot, I still have stress. I'm really worried. I have a lot of problems, but I manage my job successfully. It is my personal life that is affected by the stress. Again, I'm afraid that in the end I will get sick and will have to pay the price for this terrible stress I'm going through. I'm in AA, but I haven't had any alcohol and I haven't done drugs for the last five years. When I stopped drinking, my life changed. The alcohol in some way relaxed me and now that I don't have it, it has complicated my life.

BK: Okay.

C: Lately, I went through two events that stressed me a lot, so I took a trip. I left for four or five days and then came back. Now I feel better.

BK: A few minutes ago, at the moment when you first sat down, a very strange question popped into my mind. When that question came into my mind, all I could do was think of it. I wondered whether I should ask this question, because it's probably a crazy question. But because it popped in my mind and would not leave, I know that I must ask it. It may be a question that's hiding another question. I don't know what the question means. The question that came to my mind, the one I wanted to ask you is this: Have you ever seen a ghost?

C: I think it's a good question. I remember when I was very young. During my childhood I saw strange things. I experienced strange things, but it was such a long time ago. I'm still a little bit confused about whether they really happened or not. I thought I saw a ghost. I have developed a kind of defense about those strong and strange experiences. I have erased them from my mind as if they had never happened. I realize there are some things that I have erased along the years . . . There is one more thing—when I'm sound asleep I feel like a different energy comes into me and won't let me wake up. That has happened to me on several occasions. When I'm very tired this happens to me, and I'm very sensitive to certain circumstances and certain people, and certain energies as well.

BK: I don't think your life has anything to do with stress, nothing to do with stress at all. This is not stress.

C: What is it then?

BK: I think you are frozen.

C: Scared?

BK: I think that from the time when you saw whatever you think you saw or didn't see, you froze. When I first saw you sit down, I saw someone very still and almost frozen. As you described all the stress and the reactions you have to it, I felt like I was observing a person seeing a ghost. When someone sees a ghost, you get a frozen response that feels tight.

C: Yes, I understand. I feel that way.

BK: I would guess that you are a living puzzle that many doctors, experts, and therapists cannot understand because everything that should work with stress does not work with you. This is because it's not stress.

C: It's fear.

BK: I don't know. You're a man who saw a ghost. I don't know that anyone has told you how to live with that fact.

C: No.

BK: Not everybody has seen a ghost or sees or experiences weird things. Do you have good intuition?

C: Intuition? Regarding what?

BK: Do you ever get a special feeling about the way things are going to be?

C: Yes. It happened to me many years ago. In 1993 I had a best friend who invited me to spend a weekend in Monterrey. He was gay and he had a boyfriend. While I was in his house I had a very strong dream where this boy came in and killed us both. I woke up very upset and I told my friend the dream. I warned him to be careful with that boy because I didn't feel he was a safe person. He told me not to worry because he had him under control. He said that his boyfriend was very young and out of control, but there was no problem. Fifteen days later that boy killed my friend. He stabbed him 37 times and my friend's family asked me to claim the body. What I saw was terrible. It coincided with the previous dream and that had a big impact on me. This has happened to me on other occasions when the things I dream come true. However, this one was very unpleasant. I actually felt a little guilty because I think I should have insisted more on my friend taking me seriously. Yes, I have a special intuition. It also happens to me in business when I see problems coming. I wake up early in the morning and start having ideas and premonitions about what is going to happen. Sometimes I like it, but sometimes it bothers me.

BK: This has nothing to do with stress. Let's take the idea of stress and say, "Bye, bye. No stress." You are a man who sees ghosts and somehow this has been a blessing. But it's also been something that you have been stuck in knowing what to do with it. You are frozen in relationship to that kind of experience. It doesn't matter when you run away from things. All the things you try to do to deal with this situation don't matter, because this gift keeps visiting you—this ghost-like gift. Now I'm wondering about your intuition. If your intuition now talked to me, I would want you to not think, but only allow your intuition to communicate. I'm talking only to your intuition. I'm asking your intuition about when you were young and saw a ghost. Who does your intuition think was the ghost?

C: I don't know. It's a good question. When you asked that question, I felt something moving in my upper chest. There is a kind of emptiness there, but I don't know what is going on. I think that maybe it was not just one ghost that I experienced. Maybe there have been more, but I don't know. This is the thing: I'm afraid of contacting that part of myself. There's a terrible fear inside me and this is a part of that fear. After I stopped drinking and was part of the AA program, I complied with the 12-step program and I have been able to view my defects. I have realized that I can be very scared about some things and that fear paralyzes me. I have noticed this. Maybe I try to fly from that part of me. I run away from getting in touch with my intuition. Yes, it is a gift, but I am scared of it. I don't know how to manage it and in some way the unknown makes me scared.

BK: Your amazing life has this special gift and inner talent that you are afraid of using because you fear what you might experience. You fear experiencing a mysterious thing and this keeps you frozen. All the things you try to do, including drinking, are simply ways of running away from this thing you fear, and it has you frozen. When this thing comes to you, you feel it in your body. Your body then says, "No, I don't want to feel it." It then turns you into a frozen solid wall. All this makes so much sense. What an amazing, extraordinary being you are, to have this kind of gift and to be so humble and say, "It can't possibly be me who has this gift. I am not worthy of this gift." You then try to prove to yourself that you are not worthy of such a big good gift.

C: It's possible. I thought it was fear. I don't know.

BK: I'm having another weird thought in my mind. I see you hanging a flag in your bedroom. It's like the flag of a ship, but it hangs from your bedroom ceiling. Maybe it's a solid color, perhaps it's red, or maybe it's another color. I see you putting a flag in your bedroom that enables you to say, "I'm going to sail wherever the wind takes me and not stand still any more." I don't know why I'm telling you this. I'm just seeing this in my mind. It's a crazy thought. It's an interesting way to get your life moving. Put up a flag and declare you are going to be carried somewhere by the wind, instead of resisting.

C: In some way it's what I've been trying to do today. Even the AA program asks that I let myself go. There are some things which I cannot control, that are beyond me, and which I have to let the Higher Power be in charge. This is what I have tried to put into practice during the last couple of years and it has given me more peace. Sometimes, however, I feel afraid to know where this can lead.

BK: How many people know about this secret side of you?

C: Very few. My family knows something about it because they have been involved with this type of thing. We have many clairvoyants. From both sides of my family there are people who were and are involved with that part of magical thinking. My family believes in spiritualism, reincarnation, and traditional magic.

BK: Do they know as much about you that you shared with me today? Do they know what you told me? About your dream and about the experiences you've had since you were a child?

C: No, not all. They know some things, but they see it as something normal, as the family's legacy. But none of us has had the desire to develop it or to get more involved.

BK: What I think, in spite of your being so quiet about the secret of your life, is that your whole life is about struggling how to handle this gift. Everything, from your efforts to handle stress to your drinking, are inseparable from struggling with how to handle your special gift. You make your life secret. You are so successful with this secret that you have become a ghost to the world. Nobody sees this important part of you. It's invisible like a ghost. In some way, you've become a ghost. And understandably so. Because I'm sure if your parents, and your family knew all about what went on with you, they would say that you must do more of this. They would see this as the family legacy, as your destiny. They would want you to change your life and follow this as a special calling.

C: Do you believe that this is part of my destiny? Should I get more involved and develop this gift?

BK: I don't think about these things. I prefer listening to my intuition because these magical things cannot be understood by the mind. I just sat down with you and heard a voice immediately tell me, "This man has seen a ghost." Then later my imagination saw you putting up a flag in your bedroom and heard you saying, "I'm ready to move on with my life." Now I actually see and hear that you have become a ghost and I also remember that I'm speaking to a lawyer. That's miraculous. Who would think that a lawyer has seen a ghost and is a ghost? That's amazing. I think that there are more satisfying ways to deal with your secret, more enjoyable ways of handling your secret gift, than acting like you've just seen a ghost and clenching up into a tense frozen posture. You even dress like a ghost. You're wearing all white. You really are a ghost. (*There is laughter. Brad points to Carlos's necklace.*) What is this?

C: It's a Chinese symbol for love. This is the way you write love in Chinese.

BK: Maybe you saw a love ghost. That's what I wonder about. It seems to me like some love ghost came visiting you.

C: The microphone is out... (*The sound system suddenly stopped working.*)

BK: I think the ghost took away the microphone.

C: I thought the same.

BK: Perhaps they like to mess with electrical things. I said I think you...

C: You said I probably had seen a love ghost because it had touched this part of me (*pointing to his heart*), and that's why my chest feels funny when I think about these things. I thought that I probably have seen a love ghost. That was when the mic turned off.

BK: Some people say there are no coincidences. (*laughter*) I'm going to propose that it's wise to assume that you saw a love ghost because of what just happened. Perhaps there's nothing more to say.

C: Yes, it was amazing.

BK: Maybe a love ghost has been after you.

C: Maybe.

BK: Would you consider hanging a flag in your bedroom? It can be a little flag or a big flag. It can be a piece of colored cloth.

C: Many colors?

BK: It's your choice. What do you see? What do you feel? What does your gift tell you?

C: I see only one color and it is like wine. It is a red color, a burgundy. That is the color I see. I imagine the flag that way.

BK: That's the flag I see. We must know the same ghost.

C: I think so.

BK: Now the ghost flag can announce that you are going to get on board the love boat. (*laughter*)

C: Let's hope so.

BK: Yes. From time to time, it must be complicated to shut down all of your body because the love ghost loves you. . .

C: Yes, it's difficult.

BK: Because a love ghost comes with love, those ghosts you met as a boy weren't really scary. Their love was good. But now, all these years later, you have things a bit mixed up. Whenever you feel love coming, you feel like it's a ghost coming your way.

C: Probably it is.

BK: Put up your flag – the flag that honors love.

C: I will put it up.

BK: Say to yourself, "I'm on board the love boat." There's no reason to be scared of a love ghost anymore, because you've also become a love ghost. When that ghost comes again, you should say, "Hello, nice to see another ghost." I'm teasing you. No, I'm not. There's a truth here. I think your life has been keeping you on the shore, waiting for the boat to leave. It's interesting that you go away for a little bit and come back. It's almost like a practice or dress rehearsal to get yourself ready to move to be free to travel. I don't mean geographical travel. I mean the beating movement in your heart, the heartbeat boat that can take you to places, on journeys to the many ways that invisible love can be present. Yes, love is invisible. Love is a ghost. The capacity that you have for your body to experience life and love is huge and this is good.

C: It's possible.

BK: Are you ready to get on the boat? You've waited long enough. Raise your flag.

C: Okay.

BK: It will be nice. Will you do this? Will you hang a flag, a burgundy flag in your room? You promise?

C: I promise.

BK: Are you sure?

C: I promise.

BK: Now I see your flag hanging. Every night before you go to bed, maybe you should say, "Bon voyage" before you go to sleep. You're ready for life itself to move through your life and take you somewhere. You're ready to meet the invisible magic, the ghost of love. Ghost, we ask that you come as a wind. Blow the ship's sails. Tight body, go away. Sailing wind, take this man away on a journey to love. Do you know how to blow air?

C: Yes. (*laughing*)

BK: Blow a big puff like this. It's good for you. From this day on, the minute you think you might see or feel a ghost or have a strange feeling, it's good to know how to make a big wind.

C: Okay. I will do it!

BK: Bon voyage. If you try right now you will see what happens to your body when you blow a wind. Make the biggest breath you can and blow so hard that it makes you tremble. Try it and be surprised. Try it with me. (*Carlos and Brad each blow a big puff of air and tremble.*) Feel that? Amazing, right? I will tell you a little secret that comes from Africa. It's what the healers from some of the old tribes know. If there is ever something out there that you are uncertain about and fear, there is no need to say any magic words. There is no need to do anything except blow with all your might.

C: This is amazing. I felt something strong when you blew. I felt the energy when you blew. It was a lot of energy.

BK: It's because you feel things. We are both men ghosts. We are men who will never quite understand why the ghost of love comes to us, wanting to move us. It is a beautiful thing and a frightening thing. It is our gift and our curse. We are ghosts, but if you hoist your flag every night and say "Bon voyage," everything will be okay.

C: Okay.

BK: I think that you came here today to teach all these therapists about some extraordinary things they would otherwise never know anything about. You are an invisible man carrying ghost love, and holding other teachings, yet to be known. You can provide guidance and help to others through law, and through relationships, and through all the many ways you can touch both the mind and heart. You are not stressed. You are shipwrecked. All you have to do is get a little flag and know that your ship has come in. Always say, "Bon voyage." I think it would be nice for you to purchase a little suitcase and call it a spiritual suitcase. This suitcase shall hold things that are close to your heart. If you're at a store and you see a card that says a wonderful thing about love and it touches you, buy it and put it in your suitcase. Every time you collect something from one of your journeys of the heart, put it inside this spiritual suitcase. Please know that I feel your energy too. It's good that you've come today.

C: Thank you for seeing me.

BK: You can go everywhere your heart calls, doing so now with a new wind and a new flag and a readiness to go forward, welcoming all the surprising and extraordinary ways life is rich and complex. You have earned the right to get on board the ship. You have waited long enough. You paid all the dues. Though you've tried every way to run away from these things, they will continue coming to you. Now it will be a more interesting life because you will be on the boat, moving with the wind. Inside all the wind, carrying the wind, being the wind, being the heart, being the love, being the invisible presence of all the magic your family on both sides has waited for someone to carry into the world without fear, for the sake of the whole family's destiny and legacy. What an amazing chapter you've come to in your life. Bon voyage.

C: Thank you.

Seeing a Ghost

***

Therapists can also benefit from hoisting a flag in their office, saying out loud before a session, "I am ready to go on a journey. My ship wants to take me somewhere." Blowing a big puff of air can help release whatever holds back your creative movement. Blow the wind and drop the sails. Let the wind of a turning wheel of interactive circularity take you to a magical moment. There you will be reminded that therapy is not unlike a boat that needs a hoisted flag that announces to the world that you are at sea.

A model ship seldom gets to sea. It sits on a desk or bookshelf, sometimes next to the textbooks that prescribe models of therapy. Get onboard an authentic ship, one that is in the deep waters. Feel the currents below and the winds above. Between these eddies is something invisible that grabs hold of a vessel and takes it far. Cultivate the practice of seeing your work as requiring the utterance of a bon voyage. Know that you are on board the same ship as your clients. All of you are there for a remarkable trip. Get out of the way and let the creative wind do its job.

Why not pack a small suitcase as well? It can be a cigar box if you wish. Every time you experience a quotation that inspires you to feel a current or breeze of creativity, write it down and pack it away in your therapy suitcase. Be on the lookout for inspiring things to say. Hunt them like a pirate at sea. They are therapeutic gold and can someday turn your small suitcase into a treasure chest. Feel free to open it during a session and pull out a nugget to share with a client.

Don't forget to keep a compass of circular therapeutics nearby. Change the directions on it to read:

N: no interpretation
E: ecstatic rhapsodic expression
S: ship on a sea of interactivity
W: wind that sets your therapy free and brings it home to a healing heart

Remember Carlos and the ghost he saw and became. Maybe you saw, heard, or felt a ghost as well. It may have frozen you in a model that claims authority over your imagination, implying that you aren't ready to be at sea. Now that you know what all that is about, raise your flag and get back on course. Thank the ghost that isn't seen, while seeing the wind as your friend. Your heart has a passport and it's ready to go. Step on board and say, "Ready, set, go; the wind is ready to blow!"

11. The Water that Changed Color

In this session a father and his teenage son, Sam, come to discuss the challenges associated with the fact that they have not seen one another for most of their lives. They were separated due to an unfriendly divorce when the boy was a child in preschool. The father moved away and spent years heartbroken due to the loss of his only son. Now the father hoped to mend the bond that was previously broken. Sam had gotten into trouble for anger issues at school, and his mom asked his father, who now lived in the same town, to bring him to therapy.

At first, Brad only listened to them talk about their situation with their therapist, while observing behind a one-way mirror at a university clinic. When asked to describe his relationship with Sam, the father said it was "a little standoffish," so he doesn't try to "crowd him." The father further responded: "I just want to be with him and do things with him. I have that mindset of wanting to catch up for the ten years that I wasn't around him. I want to be his dad and his best friend, but I'm not trying to rush him. All I've had for the last ten years is a phone call. We are starting at ground zero. I feel like a stranger."

Sam nonchalantly said that "things are all right" since they had been reunited that month. When their therapist asked them what they wanted to work on in the session, Sam responded, "Whatever floats your boat, dude." His father then answered, "I'd like Sam to get a better understanding of me. I just feel like a stranger."

Sam was then asked about "the anger that everybody is talking about" and whether "everyone is overreacting." He responded, "They ain't overreacting, I promise you. I would not lie to you. I don't lie anymore. I gave up lying because it resulted in my getting grounded. That's why I ditched it. Plus I wouldn't lie to you. You're cool." The therapist brought up what happened with the previous week's session when his mother had been with him. "You know, your mom talked about your screaming at the house. Tell me more about 'the lava bed of anger within you,' as she called it."

Sam explained that he was frustrated by all the running around he had to do. He said someone always wanted him to go somewhere—school, church, a restaurant, a friend's house, and on and on. He would rather be playing his video games.

Brad entered the room and greeted Sam and his father.

BK: I just heard a little bit of your conversation, and what impressed me was something that Sam said. It's something you don't hear young men say very often. He said, "I don't lie anymore." That's awesome. It shows that you're at least trying. It's important to have a principle in your life. I was also struck by the idea that there must be a lot of emotion underneath you guys because you had a separation that wasn't something you chose. It's an emptiness that is held in a space where something is always going to be bubbling. You might mess with it and not want it to come forth in a certain kind of way, but then it comes out in a different kind of way. I want to ask you, Dad—and I say it as a father who understands this special father-son bond—do you know that when Sam grows up, you will still feel this bond? It will always be there with your kid.

Dad: Yep.

BK: Dad will always be stupid, you know. You'll find this out for yourself when you get older and have a kid. Sons will always have a part of them that thinks that Dad is dumb. That's the way it works. I want to ask you a question that is a big question. God forbid, what if something happened—and we certainly don't want this to happen—what if you never saw your father again? What if this is the last time you will ever see him? I wonder what you would want him to hear from you. What would you want to say to him? Because you never know; things happen. That's one thing I've learned in my elder years is that just when you think things are always going to be a particular way, something may happen. But you've already learned that lesson. You already know that you can't always assume that people are going to be there forever. But what if something unexpected happened and you never ever saw your father again? What would you like to tell him?

Sam: I would want to tell him that I honestly love him.

BK: Tell him that now.

S: I do honestly love you, Dad. I am right here.

D: (*with tears*) I believe you.

BK: Have you ever had a dream or woke up in the middle of the night over the past years and wished you could say that kind of thing to him. Did you ever feel that?

S: Yeah.

BK: It always touches your heart, doesn't it? (*Brad now turns and looks at Dad*) Did you hear what he just said?

D: Uh-huh.

BK: He's dreamed about you and dreamed about saying that to you. I know he woke up weeping too. I bet you had the same experience, Dad.

D: Yes.

BK: Why don't you give each other a hug? It's a good thing for men to hug.

(*Sam flies out of his chair and gives his dad a big hug.*)

BK: We take life for granted, and we forget to say those kinds of things when we feel it. You each have been dreaming each other. Do you know what that means? It means you were never separate from one another. *(Brad turns to their therapist and talks to him.)* They were never separate. Their hearts were right next to each other. No matter how far away they were, they were dreaming, longing, and feeling each other. Their feelings may have been realized more intensely than those young boys who lived with their dads all the time. Those boys often take their relationship for granted. But these two were separate, so they couldn't take their relationship for granted. Their situation woke up a feeling inside of them that not all dads and their sons allow themselves to feel.

(Brad then turns to Sam and his Dad and continues.) What you showed me today tells me that you didn't take your love for granted. You felt it, and now when you are physically together, it must be sort of weird because you were so close when you were apart.

D: Uh-huh.

BK: This is like another reality. You already shared tenderness for one another in your private moments and in your dreams. But now here you are facing one another. I'm happy you brought your feelings here today and honestly expressed them, because you just never know what might happen.

D: Man, that is right on the money.

BK: Life is a mystery. We'll never fully understand the reasons why you weren't able to live physically side by side. But we do know that it is a great mystery that life gave you that heartfelt connection. Fathers and sons usually put a shell around their hearts, and some fathers and sons live their whole lives never experiencing what you just said to one another. It's hard to believe, but it's true. I've seen old men who were sad because they'd never said that to their father. I'm feeling something in my heart, and I am going to allow some words to come forth for both of you. You're both very lucky. Every human being is like a volcano with all kinds of emotions inside. Unfortunately, we usually put a cap on it and bottle it all up. Then we pretend that we don't have any emotions. But this wasn't so for you guys even when you were separated. You'd go to sleep, and whoosh—all that love and longing and missing would just come out. That's amazing because it means you're both going to be open and tender, not only to each other but to all of your life. I assume that it's such a powerful experience that when it comes up, it almost overcomes you. It's almost too much to handle sometimes. It hurts to love and long for your father that much. It hurts to love and long for your son that much. You almost wish that it would stay inside the volcano. Do you understand what I'm saying?

S: Yes, sir.

D: Yes.

BK: You two have been opened by life. Not all men have been opened. A lot of men have so much armor around their heart that it's uncertain to others whether they really feel anything. But I know something about you two. You both have felt emotions as powerfully and as deeply as is possible for a human being to experience. Right? You know it because you woke up in the middle of the night feeling that longing, loving, and wanting of your father. If it had been any more powerful, it would have felt like it was more than you could take. It's so interesting to find both a father and a son who have been opened. I am not even sure why I'm saying this, but I feel that maybe you were chosen to be opened in this powerful way. Do you know what I mean?

(*Both Sam and his dad nod in agreement.*)

BK: This makes you different and special because here sits a father and son who are both opened. Of course it comes with some interesting side effects. It means other kinds of emotions can flow out much more easily too. So, Sam, when you get annoyed, all that emotion knows how to shoot right up.

(*Now Brad turns to Sam's dad.*) When he feels that he's been wronged, misunderstood, that things aren't rational, when he's been put in a position that he shouldn't be in, then his volcanic fire gets stirred and spews forth, but for him it probably feels natural to shoot a whole lot of fire. A young man who has been opened to have the flow of gentle love also finds that the flow of angry fire comes easily too. One doesn't come without the other. You see, he's going to feel strongly about everything.

D: Yes, that's right.

BK: I bet you have felt the anger too about how life has wronged you and about how things didn't work out the way you wanted. At times it may feel like a crazy rage. You just want to lift your car off the ground and throw it across the road and have it land somewhere.

D: Yep!

BK: So you both have those two things opened. You have felt the flow of love and the flow of anger. I'm wondering what other things have flowed from you. Have you also been able to find the deep, wild, and crazy, ridiculous laughter that is within you? Do you guys know if you've had that one flow?

S: Oh yeah, we do.

BK: Do you ever start laughing so hard that you can't stop laughing?

S: There was one of them today. He cracked me up.

BK: Really? That's awesome. That's very impressive.

D: I have laughed so hard that I'm crying!

BK: Wow! You guys are triply opened.

D: Yep!

BK: I thought that maybe you were so serious from the other heavy kind of openings that you might have missed this light one, but you got this one too. That's great. So when you get together, do you ever bring this silliness into the world? I ask because the world doesn't give a whole lot of space for being stupid, silly, ridiculous, and a little crazy. You know what I mean? Everybody is too serious. Everything at school is too serious. Since you guys are already opened, you don't need to do the stuff that most fathers and sons need to do. You don't need to mess around with seeing whether you can open your hearts and express your love because you've been doing that for all these years. You both made that clear. You also know how to shoot some volcanic fire if the circumstances elicit it. I'm sure you'll learn how to manage all that. A lot of dads have to take their kids out and teach them how to take care of themselves. It seems he already has that opened, though it's a little clumsy right now. It will smooth itself out. I think you need to spend more time together exploring how to be two funny guys: two wild and crazy guys. I don't know exactly what that means. Maybe it means checking out a movie that is most likely to tickle you. Or maybe you become merry tricksters. Dad, were you ever a guy who pulled practical jokes and stunts?

S: I do that all the time.

D: I have done some stunts. I had a good teacher. That was my father.

(*At this point Brad turns to their therapist and gives some direction.*) I think you should have a little talk with them about how they can turn themselves into rascals and unique characters. Ask them to find some ways to tickle themselves when they are together. Please talk about it while I take a little break. I'll watch you from behind the one-way mirror. OK, you guys are awesome. I'll be right back.

(*Brad goes back to the observing room.*)

D: Wow! That was heavy. It was deep.

S: It made an impact. It's very hard to make an impact on me.

They discussed whether they could do something wild and crazy, but to the therapist's surprise, Sam offered a caution. "Well, we don't want to do anything too crazy." That was Brad's cue to reenter.

BK: You two are way too serious.

D: I know.

BK: You know you don't need to be that serious anymore. Seriously. You already know everything you need to know: Your son loves you. He woke up in the middle of the night and felt the love so intensely that he would sob, and you felt the same. You guys have a bond that's going to last forever. We've heard you both say it and express it today. I don't think you ever need to talk about it again. From this moment on remind yourself of this fact: you know what some fathers never know, and you know it in a way that some fathers would give anything to experience. They would give away all the money they ever earned to experience what your son has expressed and felt for you. Do you get that?

D: Yes, I do.

BK: Will you accept it?

D: Yes.

BK: Let's just say adios to having to worry about it.

D: Yes.

(Note: When Brad went behind the mirror, he took all the objects that were sitting on a desk—a red candle, a foam cup, some transparent tape, and two lollipops. Without thinking he tied most of those things together and entered the room, held up the lollipop, and made an announcement).

BK: Here's a lollipop. I want to see more lollipop in your life.

(Brad then presented what he had thrown together for them. It was a red candle that had a white foam cup hanging from its middle, hung by strips of tape. The cup was half-filled with water.)

BK: I want to see you guys be a little crazy with me now. Why in the world would a therapist give you something like this? You know it's a red candle and it has a wick. It hasn't yet been lit, but it could be lit and then we'd have a fire. This candle has a cup attached to it with a little water, and it's held by sticky tape that may hold or not hold. Now that's crazy isn't it? When you walked in today, you didn't expect that, did you?

(The father and son both look stunned by the absurd presentation of a red candle that holds a suspended cup of water.)

BK: You are probably asking, what in the world are we going to do with that? I'm going to hand this thing to you now. Sam, hold one end of the candle while Dad holds the other end.

(At this moment the father and son hold the ends of a candlestick. They keep it level because a half-full cup of water was hanging from the middle of the stick.)

BK: Now I want you two to take a pledge. You two will declare to the world that you are going to be a father and son unlike anything anyone has ever seen. Do you agree?

(*They both say in unison, "Yes."*)

BK: You will dedicate yourself to promoting silliness in every possible opportunity that comes your way.

(*They both nod.*)

BK: You, Dad, will devote yourself to making him laugh so hard that it will hurt. Yes?

D: Yes.

BK: And you, Sam, will devote yourself to making Dad laugh so hard it will hurt.

S: Yes!

BK: Somehow, this is going to make another opening not only within each of you but with others you two meet in the world. This will surprise you. You might even wake up one night with a dream that you've been laughing so hard that you fell out of the bed and are rolling on the floor. That would be something! Wouldn't that be something?

D: OK, Son, are you up for it?

S: Yes! (*Sam nods enthusiastically.*)

BK: Why continue looking for what you've always had? Why get angry over that which you already can handle? You know how to handle everything. You have what you need and what you want. You, Dad, have what he wants. You, Sam, have what he wants. It's all come down on you like a shower of blessings. You have everything. You just haven't gotten this in your mind. Do you know what I'm saying?

D & S: Yes.

BK: You two are amazing. I want to jump up and down and be a cheerleader and say, "Go out there and show the world what is possible."

D: Yes!

BK: Show them what a dad and son can do besides all the talk you might hear in a psychotherapy clinic. Forget all that. Don't pay attention to any of this nonsense. You guys have enough therapy. You've got each other. You hold each other's hearts. You've got each other in terms of knowing how to take care of what matters most. You know how to work yourself up if you need protection. When you don't need to do that, you don't need to do that. What is important now is for you to learn to be funnier.

(*Brad points to the water that was suspended under the red candle.*)

BK: Maybe that's not water. Maybe it's nitroglycerin. Wouldn't that be something?

D: We wouldn't want to light the candle then. Or maybe we do want to light the candle and see what happens.

S: That's crazy; we don't want to light it.

BK: Very interesting. Maybe it's holy water and if you put your finger in it, you'll be blessed for life. Maybe you'll be blessed in a way that will shock both of you. You might find that you won't be able to stop laughing. Perhaps you better not do that. (*pause*) I am going to ask you each to touch the water now. It's important. Touch the water.

(*Dad carefully sticks his finger into the water. He then looks at Sam and leans his head forward to gesture that it is Sam's turn.*)

S: Who, me?

D: Yes.

(*Sam slowly and carefully sticks his finger into the water. As he does so, Brad chants.*)

BK: Walk on water, walk on water. Yes, holy water, yes.

D: I say light the candle.

BK: Hey, look where the wick is pointing. Look whose end has the wick.
  (*The wick is near Sam.*)

S: Dad, I know you have a lighter.

(*Dad pulls out a lighter and lights the candlewick. They now hold a candle that is lit.*)

BK: I am going to propose that no one in the history of the world has ever done what the two of you are doing right now. I will bet everything that a father and son have never held a hot candle with a wick

The Water that Changed Color   *219*

pointed toward a son who was sitting there ready to be lit.

(*Brad reaches over and gives the cup a little push. It starts swinging back and forth.*)

BK: These men have baptized the tips of their fingers and walked upon this water. Now they are sitting here wondering what in the world this is doing to them, but of course it doesn't have to mean a thing—it can just be an unexpected moment that is the beginning of more unexpected moments. I can just see them twenty years from now—maybe they will be at a ballgame or at home watching a movie and they will say, "Remember the time we held that candle and swinging cup?"

(*Both Sam and his Dad start laughing,* "Yeah!")

BK: Let's cover up what is happening here. I think we can make this even more mysterious if we set it up so nobody can really see what is going on between the two of you.

(*Brad takes some tissues and covers both of their hands as they hold the candle and cup.*)

BK: Now no one can ever see that you are holding each other's hands, side by side with the help of a lit stick that bridges the distance. Like before, this connection you have is so intense that it is red hot. It shows your hearts are wide open.

(*Dad and Sam nod their heads and agree.*)

BK: (*in an hypnotic tone*) I see what has happened to you. Every once in a while, a fire in their world would overcome them, and it filled their cup with tears. (*Brad points to the water in the cup.*) Sometimes this fire became hot and angry so that someone needed to take a little water and . . . (*At this moment Brad slaps the cup so it spills some water.*) Bam! Just like that, it helps that little fire get extinguished.

D: That makes a lot of sense.

BK: Weird, isn't it?

S: That does make a lot of sense.

BK: Here are two men with an invisible relationship that they can feel and hold onto. These two men have taken a special pledge today. They have promised they are going to do something together that is weird and funny. They might even go into their backyard and sing a song to a squirrel.

(*Everyone starts laughing, but the burning red candle and cup of water are still in their hands.*)

BK: Do you two have pet names for each other?

S: I have a nickname from everyone at school. It is Weenie.

(*BK points to the stick they were holding.*)

BK: There it is, there it is. It's a red hot dog.

S: If I'm the weenie, what is Dad?

D: I'm the bun. We're the weenie and the bun.

BK: I love that! You guys, Weenie and Bun, make one interesting hot dog! You should choose a song as your anthem.

S: Yeah, that's cool.

BK: You should not hold anything back. Do as many things as you can that will be spectacular for the world. You might even someday write a book about your new partnership. It could happen.

(*Sam peeks under the Kleenex to look at the cup of water. He looks quite surprised.*)

BK: Whoa, Sam. Is anything happening under there?

S: The water is a different color.

BK: Wow! It changed color.

D: (*lifting the Kleenex*) Let me look.

BK: The mind is an interesting thing.

S: (*looking at his dad*) Don't you think it has changed color? (*Dad shakes his head with uncertainty.*) It did, man! The water changed color!

(*Brad gives each of them a lollipop and invites them to open it and put it in their mouth.*)

BK: Look at these guys with those sticks coming out of their mouths. What in the world are they holding? These two guys are funny!

(*Someone knocks on the door. It is the clinic director who wants to take a Polaroid photograph of the father and son holding the lit red candle with the attached water that may have changed color, doing so while* they have lollipops in their mouths.)

BK: Yes! We want to record this historical moment.

D: (*Dad pulls off the tissue so the whole setup can be seen.*) This doesn't need to be covered anymore.

BK: Yes, that's right. You know your dad just took that cover off. Do you know what that means? It means that you two are being unveiled. You are now set free in the world as partners ready to have some crazy wild adventures. (*Their photograph is taken.*) Someday I will pick up a newspaper and see a photograph that looks like this one or I will see the news on television and find that they have become wild and crazy adventurers. They will take vacations together and enjoy surprise visits to roadside diners. They will do all this just so they can tell other fathers and sons that they need to lighten up. The headline will say, "Weenie and Bun Take Their Hot Dog Stunts across America."

(*Brad hands them the Polaroid photograph that has been taken of them.*) I want you to take this with you as a reminder that you have always been holding onto each other and it's been a heart-to-heart connection. No matter how much heat life gives you, there is always a cup of water underneath to do what it needs to do.

BK: (*stands up to shake their hands*) You guys are amazing.

S: It has been interesting to meet you.

BK: It was really nice to meet you, Sam.

S: I am glad that I got chosen.

BK: I feel it too, Sam. You were chosen to have a remarkable life because nothing like this happens unless it is meant to happen. (*Brad shakes Dad's hand.*) I am so glad I got to meet you. It is awesome isn't it?

D: Oh yes, it is!

(*Everyone in the room hugs one another.*)

BK: Hey guys, the world needs us. They need to see this because the world has gotten too heavy. Everyone needs to lighten up. Go show them how. Have a great life. I expect it.

***

Sam and his dad teach us that all of us already have what we think is missing. In their case, it was their love and caring for one another. What they needed more of was to exercise some simple fun. Though being silly was already a part of their everyday, it needed to be given more importance. Did the water change color? The answer is found in a more fascinating question: did their relationship change? In the beginning an adolescent sat with a man who felt like a stranger. At the end, they were two buddies, Weenie and Bun, ready to go on some exciting adventures.

Bring more lightheartedness to your sessions and find that this makes it easier for the transformative light to be seen. Utilize whatever is in front of you, even if it includes some junk that was left on a table. Everything you need is right in front of you. Reach out and hold onto it. Do so while allowing the inspiration of a circular interaction to improvise what will happen next. Do so to be caught inside a movement that gives less importance to having to understand in order to know how to act. Act in order to allow change to happen, with or without any glimpse of an understanding. In this way, you might get tickled as you find how effortless it is to help bring forth the beacon that brings us all home.

INTERLUDE

What must a therapist know to become a healer?

What does a healer forget in order to escape the limitations of therapy?

Is there some "not knowing" going on here?

And some not "not knowing"?

Would it matter if you knew?

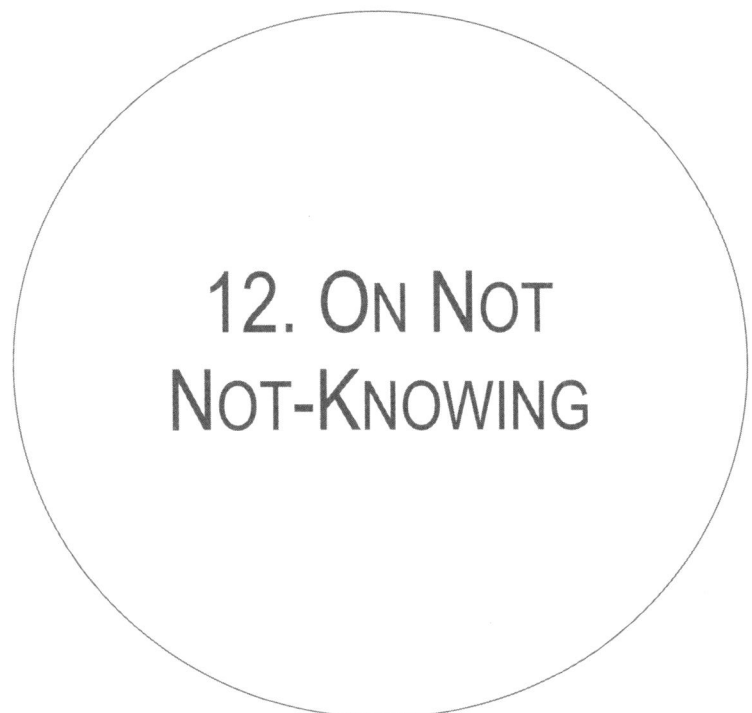

12. ON NOT NOT-KNOWING

Here we wish to teach that it is sometimes wise to say less on matters concerning not knowing. Not saying is often the best teacher of not knowing. We illustrate with a story:

Once upon a time a healer was asked by a sincere therapist, "Please heal my chattering mind." The healer responded with a story:
> Once upon a time a poet was asked by a sincere healer, "Please give me words to say when I don't know what to say." The poet responded with three little words, "No to know."

Before there was Zen, a master of Zen was asked by a therapist, healer, and a poet, "Please give us a wise story." She responded with a nap, until all three fell asleep watching the master sleep. In their dreams a song was heard by all:
> On the silent stage is found the sound.
> Dream a song so no tale is told.
> No other way can release the hold.

INTERLUDE

On the road again, our well-storied client finally got her chance to speak at a conference of therapists. Everyone wondered what she would say. She began by acknowledging that there will always be strict judges, accurate stenographers, totalizing theorists, guardians of clinical models, and pious historical archivists who will point to well-worn documents and argue that they indicate a precedent for how we should act today.

She went on to caution everyone about following advice based on words uttered by those who are now dead. Life—in its present living—holds the necessary wisdom to naturally bring forth each expressive moment. As she put it, "Do not spook the living present by any past haunting. Let presence be present and allow the past to pass. Whatever is important about the past lives inside the present."

At that moment in her talk, a bee flew into an open window and buzzed around the auditorium. She stopped, pointed to the bee, and said, "The bee has come to remind us that we should remember the difference between its waggle dance and round dance. The former indicates that food is far away, while a round dance communicates that it is nearby. You already know how to waggle—you theoretically draw from what is faraway or in the past. I have been trying to teach you how to be nearer to the source, what is close at hand."

She started singing with all her might. It appeared that she was singing to the bee, for it circled around her, as they each inspired one another. She sang of all the things that can help transform a therapist into a healer. When she finished, she leaned into the microphone and whispered, "The journey from therapy to healing moves you from archive to beehive, for that which delivers the sting also brings the honey."

13. KOAN: Should Therapy Be an Archive or a Beehive?

POINTER
There are many gates to the heart of healing. The healer's gait is as wide as an ocean's heart. Searching for the mangoes that fell off the back of your cart, you will surely lose your way. Here, now—utilize this!

THE CASE
A student asked the old teacher, "How shall I draw my conclusion?"
The old man answered, "The storyteller swallows her own tale."

APPRECIATORY VERSE
A tail is swallowed with each turning,
A new tale born with every yearning.
Hiding on the shelf, even the most beautiful poem gathers dust.
What's the shelf-life of one great moment?
To answer, change!
Mother Samuel has cooked you a meal.
Please eat it.

Metalogue on the Case

Student: Are we finished?

Circular Poet: You can now either create an archive or you can create a beehive.

S: I don't understand. What does that have to do with this book?

CP: One buzzes, the other doesn't.

S: Now you are messing with me.

CP: No, I'm very serious. You should be careful around archives. They can offer a deadly sting.

S: You mean beehives, I should be careful around beehives because I'm allergic to bees.

CP: No. That is not what I mean. Archives can be deadly. I think I may be allergic to archives, but that's another conversation entirely.

S: What's wrong with archives? They are important collections of history and ideas that otherwise would be lost to future generations. If we didn't have archives so much wisdom would be lost.

CP: Yes, that is true. Archives are wonderful in that way. In all seriousness, there is nothing wrong with having an archive. It's just that I once met a man whose claim to fame was having an incredible archive of books, notes, and materials of some of the most creative and imaginative professors. It really was a wonderful archive, and there was a lot of important information in there, and lots of inspiring material.

S: Yes, I read about that archive. It sounds like a good thing that he was so invested in keeping it alive.

CP: Sure, in one sense it was great. Everyone kept inviting him to go around the world and talk about the archive and tell the stories of those great teachers.

S: What's wrong with that?

CP: Have you ever heard the story of the Buddha's attendant, Ananda?

S: Yes, at least part of it. It's said he was at the Buddha's side for over twenty years or something like that. Didn't he memorize all the Buddha's teachings?

CP: Apparently in the Buddha's time they didn't write down any of his speeches or talks, and so when the Buddha died, it was Ananda who recited the Buddha's teachings word for word so that they could then begin to record them for future generations. Ananda had listened so intently to the Buddha that he was able to recite the teachings in such a way that people could not tell whether it was he or the Buddha talking (Keizan, 2003).

S: That is impressive.

CP: Except, as impressive as that was, Ananda had never achieved enlightenment, though he did later after the Buddha died. As it says in the Buddhist archives:

> ...Ananda was fond of much hearing and therefore had still not achieved perfect enlightenment.... Truly, much hearing is an obstacle to the Way, and this is the evidence. Therefore, the *Avatamsaka Sutra* says, "Much hearing is like a poor person who counts another's treasure and hasn't a halfpenny of his own." (Keizan, 2003, p. 38)

S: Are you saying that this man with the archive is like Ananda?

CP: I'm saying that you are not the first person to notice the difference between description and embodiment.

S: It seems to be an ongoing human trap, this dizzying dance in and out of knowing and not-knowing, naming and being, narrativity and interactivity.

CP: Seems to be. The man with the archive went around sharing all these wonderful stories and videos of these transformative teachers who were formerly alive, creative, absurd, improvisational, and dynamic, but he himself was largely none of those. I mean he tried to teach others some of the wisdom those teachers held, of course, so he was better than a lot of the others who were totally lost, but he was missing the point.

S: Because he was so busy talking about the archive?

CP: He had good intentions, but you can't eat a painting of an orange.

S: Very funny.

CP: Try it yourself—it has no juice.

S: So you mean he just got all obsessed with the archive and forgot that the stories were about professors eating oranges, but this guy never ate a real orange?

CP: Yes, something like that. But if I were to say it differently, I would say that one has to be careful telling the same stories over and over again, even if they are good stories. Even if they are Buddhist sutras. Probably if those same professors in the archive were alive today, they would be changing all of the time because their wisdom was full of interactive presence and vitality. They would be alive, not as an archive, but more like a beehive, full of buzz and honey, pointing to what's funny, if...

S: Enough with the rhyming. The APA Manual says to avoid poetic language.

CP: That is why APA is boring.

S: I knew you would say that.

CP: Then I've become predictable. See? Archives are deadly.

S: And beehives have more buzz.

CP: And more honey.

S: Maybe that guy should burn the archive.

CP: Yes! Or maybe not, because the archive is a nice thing. Perhaps next time he shows up for a speech about the archive and all those amazing teachers, he should explain instead why his not talking about the archive is a better transmission of its teachings.

S: Maybe a metaphorical ceremonial burning. He could just burn one tiny letter of the archive.

CP: Great idea! And then you could send him a tiny, plastic model of a beehive with a card that says, "Here's to getting the sweet buzz back into your life!" Make sure you take him out for a celebratory beer. That might be all he needs: a good burn, a good beehive, and a good buzz!

S: It's during times like these I'm glad you are my teacher.

CP: Great, then buy me a beer.

S: Would anyone possibly consider adding this book to an archive someday?

CP: Perhaps. But you have to be a beehive before anyone will want to make an archive out of your work.

S: So, what now? Should I keep writing about circular therapeutics and a healing heart for therapy? Should I try to get a job performing circular therapeutics? Does such a job exist?

CP: I don't know if you would find it in academia. Anything is possible, but just as I am allergic to archives, academic institutions are by and large allergic to creativity. Talking about creativity will make you sound hip, but being too creative will either be threatening to the people who write about creativity, or just make you seem weird. Or there will just be no time, because of all the meetings.

S: That's depressing.

CP: I once heard about a man who was a leading cybernetic epistemologist, and then one day he dropped out of academia to go learn from healers all over the world who couldn't read.

S: Why?

CP: Mostly because he dreamed that he was supposed to, but partly because he was in love with ideas, but realized academia is not so much about great scholarship but about ego, competition, and small-mindedness. His choice was either to be what he called an "intellectual terrorist," bombing ignorance with academic papers, or become a servant of love. He chose love, which he found flowed more easily among those who had no archives. Also those people without archives were funnier and teased each other more. It's funny how he met some people in the Kalahari who have a spiritual relationship with bees—now that's something to ponder.

S: That sounds a bit like a cliché, though, to say that those with less book knowledge have more wisdom.

CP: Perhaps. But it's a cliché worth remembering for the truth it contains about what life was like before there even was a printing press.

S: Whatever happened to that guy?

CP: Which one—the archivist? He's still in the archive.

S: No, the guy who became a love servant or whatever.

CP: He had a dream that his head was on fire and he fell in love with a poet. He called her a silver trout.

S: Trout? Like the fish?

CP: The silver trout from Yeats' poem.

S: What happened to them?

CP: I heard they swim together, forever. Isn't that beautiful?

S: Yes, I think so.

CP: How about that beer? Or should we have a sazerac? I'll tell you some more tales of bees and being in love.

S: Sure, as long as we can go dancing later on.

CP: Have we become a circular poem?

S: Does a dancing bee make honey while a poet circles a line?

CP: Does a therapist become a healer when she is able to both sting and sing?

S: Only if there is sweetness encircling the hive, rather than the stench of death in an archive.

CP: You are dancing me, aren't you?

S: In the sweet honey of the academic rock, a therapist is wanting to be more than a clock. There he is, ticking away at the answers until a question stings him to jump up and say, "I'd rather dance than get stuck inside a narrative trance."

CP: Would you take a chance to lose whatever wisdom the bee can circulate by taking a glance at a book that knows it all?

S: I want to archive that question.

CP: I'm okay with that as long as you promise to burn your answer.

S: I will burn my answer if your question will take me dancing.

CP: Now my head is spinning.

S: Someday I hope you will ask me whether your heart is buzzing.

CP: It is, my dear. Shall we go home and get our fishing gear?

S: Wait, one more thing. Who is Mother Samuel?

CP: She was one of the most revered Shakers of St. Vincent, a real holy woman who was loved by many. She was known for being able to fix magical meals out of just a few simple ingredients (Keeney, 2010).

S: How did she do that? What made them magical?

CP: Mother Samuel always sang and prayed over the food while she cooked it. She poured all her love into every meal she made, so when people ate, they were nourished by more than just the food on the plate. People say she brought people to God by fixing them a meal.

S: So Mother Samuel was about helping people taste life's holy meal, rather than just the menu card?

CP: Something like that, yes. Let's go catch some fish.

S: And when we fry it up, let's remember to sing a song for Mother Samuel.

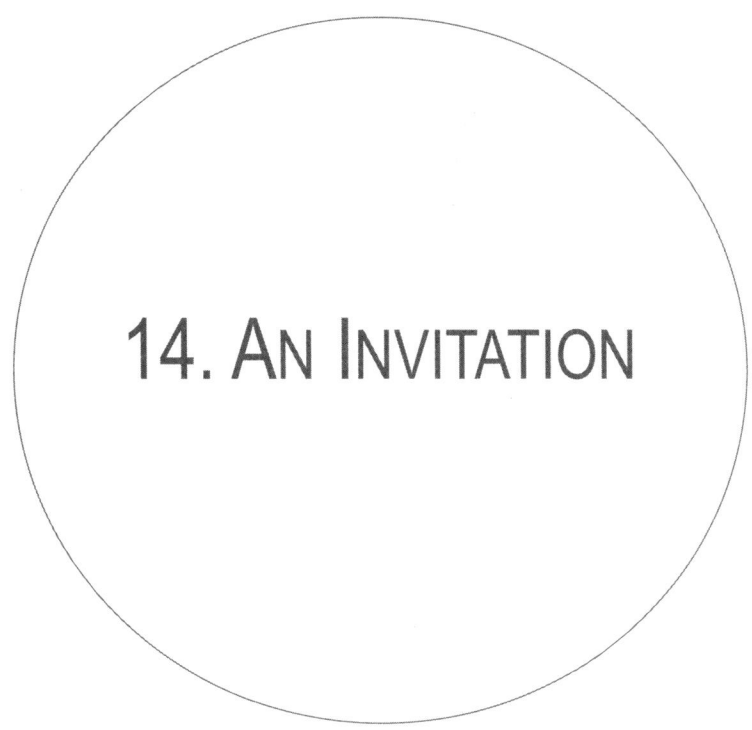

14. An Invitation

He who binds to himself a joy
Doth the winged life destroy;
But he who kisses the joy as it flies
Lives in Eternity's sun rise.
—William Blake

We shall not say that our ending holds the beginning because we feel we have not begun. Nor do we intend to ever end. Consider the word "intend" now that we have mentioned it. Throw away its "end" and you are left with three letters: "int," the beginning of the word "interactivity," the process of creation that assures a never-ending beginning.

We have given our three basic steps to becoming a therapist with a healing heart, a performer of circular therapeutics. In case you forgot, we will say them again, saying them differently in case you remember. Number one, hush little puppy. Two, move around, with an emphasis on round. And three, celebrate the change without any distracting concern about whether it has fully arrived. Of course, we never reach the end of any step, and all three are mastered if only one step is ever fully taken. Though this is a tease, it shuns any trivial way of trying to please. For your life depends on whether you pledge to stop the flood of narration and hop on board the ship that sails the sea of improvisation. Otherwise, you will not have a song, which is to say, you'll lose the art of sailing a healing heart.

We invite you to join circulus, the circus that circulates circularity. There is a lineage of those who dance the contraries—from early day sacred fools to wandering poets, singers of the blues, and postmodern cyberneticians—all of them in relationship with ancient healers and creative therapists. Each belongs to the turning that turns a ceremonial space, clinic, or theatre into a creative circularity inside the circle of life. Welcome to circular therapeutics, where therapy changes with a healing heart.

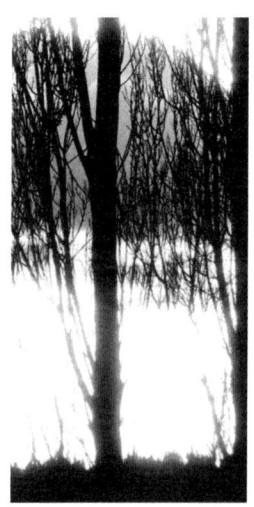

REFERENCES

Anderson, H. (1997). *Conversations, language, and possibilities: A postmodern approach to therapy.* New York, NY: Basic Books.

Anderson, H. (2007). The therapist and the postmodern therapy system: A way of being *with* others. *6th Congress of the European Family Therapy Association and 32nd Association for Family Therapy and Systemic Practice UK Conference.* October 5, 2007. Glasgow, Scotland. Retrieved from http://www.eftacim.org/doc_pdf/anderson.pdf

Bateson, G. (1972). *Steps to an ecology of mind.* Chicago, IL: University of Chicago Press.

Bateson, G. (1974). Scattered thoughts for a conference on "broken power". *CoEvolutionary Quarterly, 4,* 26-27.

Bateson, G. (2002). *Mind and nature: A necessary unity.* Cresskill, NJ: Hampton Press.

Bateson, G. & Bateson, M.C. (1987). *Angels fear: Towards an epistemology of the sacred.* New York, NY: Macmillan.

Bateson, G., Weakland, J. & Haley, J. (1976). Comments on Haley's "history". In C.E. Sluzki & D. C. Ransom, (Eds.), *Double bind: The foundation of the communicational approach to the family* (105-110). New York, NY: Grune & Stratton, Inc.

Bröcker, M. (2003). Between the lines: The part-of-the-world-position of Heinz von Foerster. *Cybernetics and Human Knowing, 10*(2), 51–65.

Charlton, N. G. (2008). *Understanding Gregory Bateson: Mind, beauty, and the sacred earth.* Albany, NY: State University of New York Press.

Clarke, B., & Hansen, M. (Eds.). (2009). *Emergence and embodiment: New essays on second-order systems theory.* Durham, NC: Duke University Press.

Cleary, T., & Cleary, J. C. (1977). *The blue cliff record.* Boston, MA: Shambhala.

Dumoulin, H. (2006). The song period: A time of maturation. In John Daido Loori (Ed.), *Sitting with koans* (pp. 17–39). Sommerville, MA: Wisdom. (Original work published 1988).

Goodchild, P. (1993). Speech and silence in the Mumonkan: An examination of use of language in light of the philosophy of Gilles Deleuze. *Philosophy east and west, 43*(1), 1–18. Retrieved from California Institute of Integral Studies Religion and Philosophy Collection Database. Available from http://www.jstor.org/stable/1399466

Harries-Jones, P. (1995). *A recursive vision: Ecological understanding and Gregory Bateson.* Toronto, CA: University of Toronto Press.

Haley, J. (1973). *Uncommon therapy.* New York, NY: W.W. Norton.

Haley. J. (1976a). *Problem solving therapy.* San Francisco: Jossey-Bass.

Haley, J. (1976b). Development of a theory: A history of a research project. In C.E. Sluzki & D. C. Ransom, (Eds.). *Double Bind: The Foundation of the Communicational Approach to the Family.* New York, NY: Grune & Stratton, Inc. pp. 59-104. Original work published in 1961.

Hoffman, L. (1993a). Beyond power and control: Towards a "second-order" family systems therapy. In Hoffman, L., *Exchanging voices: A collaborative approach to family therapy.* London, England: Karnac books. (Original article published in 1985).

Hoffman, L. (1993b). *Exchanging voices: A collaborative approach to family therapy.* London, England: Karnac books.

Hoffman, L. (2002). *Family therapy: An intimate history.* New York, NY: Norton.

Hurston, Z. N. (1997). *The sanctified church: The folklore writings of Zora Neale Hurston.* New York, NY: Marlowe & Company.

Jackson, D. (1957). The question of family homeostasis. *The Psychiatric Quarterly Supplement, 31 (part 1), 79-90.*

Jackson, D. (1961). Interactional psychotherapy. In M. Stein (Ed.), *Contemporary psychotherapies* (pp. 256–271). New York, NY: Free Press of Glenco.

Jackson, D. (1965). The study of the family. *Family Process, 4*(1), 1-20.

Jung, C. G. (1974). *Myserium coniunctionis: Collected Works, Vol. 14* (G. Adler & R. F. C. Hull, Trans.). Princeton, NJ: Princeton University Press.

Keels, B. (in press). *The Hoffman blunder: An examination of the deevolution from systemic to interpretive practice.* Unpublished doctoral dissertation.

Keeney, B. P. (1977). *On paradigmatic change: Conversations with Gregory Bateson.* Unpublished manuscript.

Keeney, B. P. (1979). Ecosystemic epistemology: An alternative paradigm for diagnosis. *Family Process, 18*, 117–133.

Keeney, B. (1982). Not pragmatics, not aesthetics. *Family Process, 21*(4), 429-434.

Keeney, B. P. (1983). *Aesthetics of change.* New York, NY: Guilford Press.

Keeney, B. P. (1991). *Improvisational therapy: A practical guide for creative clinical strategies.* New York, NY: Guilford Press.

Keeney, B. P. with G. Bateson (1996). *Conversations with Gregory Bateson.* Unpublished manuscript.

Keeney, B. (1999), *Kalahari Bushmen healers,* Philadelphia: Ringing Rocks Press.

Keeney, B. (2003), *Ropes to God: Experiencing the Bushman spiritual universe,* Philadelphia: Ringing Rocks Press.

Keeney, B. P. (2007). Batesonian epistemology, Bushman n/om-kxaosi, and rock art. *Kybernetes, 36*(7–8), 884–904.

Keeney, B. P. (2009). *The creative therapist: The art of awakening a session.* New York, NY: Routledge.

Keeney, B. P. (2010). *The Bushman way of tracking god.* New York, NY: Atria Books.

Keeney, B. P. & Ross, J. M. (1985). *Mind in therapy: Constructing systemic family therapies.* New York, NY: Basic Books.

Keeney, B. P. & Silverstein, O. (1986). *The therapeutic voice of Olga Silverstein.* New York: Guilford.

Keeney H. S. (2011). *Circular poetics: Cybernetics, Zen koans, and the art of creative transformative pedagogy* (Doctoral dissertation). Retrieved from ProQuest Dissertations and Theses (916617375).

Keeney, H. & Keeney, B. (2012a). Externalization in narrative therapy: Addressing a modernist reemergence of exorcism. *Terapia y Familia (Journal of the Mexican Association of Family Therapy).*

Keeney, H. & Keeney, B. (2012b). What is systemic about systemic therapy? Therapy models muddle embodied systemic practice. *Journal of Systemic Therapies, 31* (1), 22-37.

Keizan, J. (2003). *The record of transmitting the light: Zen master Keizan's denkoroku.* (FJ Cook, Trans.) . Sommerville, MA: Wisdom Publications.

Korzybski, A. (1994). *Science and sanity: An introduction to non-Aristotelian systems and general semantics* (5th ed.). Englewood, NJ: Institute of General Semantics.

Krippendorf, K. (2012). Book endorsement. In H. Keeney & B. Keeney, *Circular therapeutics: Giving therapy a healing heart*. Phoenix, AZ: Zeig, Tucker, & Theisen.

Kwang, W. (1997). *Open mouth, already a mistake: Talks by Zen master Wu Kwang*. Cumberland, RI: Primary Point Press.

Loori, J. D. (Ed.). (2006). *Sitting with koans: Essential writings on the practice of Zen koan introspection*. Boston, MA: Wisdom.

Maturana, H. & Varela, F. (1980). *Autopoiesis and cognition: The realization of the living*. Boston, MA: Reidel.

Maslow, A. (1964). *Religions, values, and peak-experiences*. Columbus, OH: Ohio State University Press.

McGoldrick, M., Giordano, J., & Garcia-Preto, N. (Eds.) (2005). *Ethnicity & family therapy*. New York, NY: Guilford Press. Third edition.

Minuchin, S. (1974). Families & family therapy. Cambridge, MA: Harvard University Press.

Minuchin, S. (1998). Where is the family in narrative family therapy? *Journal of Marital and Family Therapy, 24*(4), 397-403.

Miura, I. & Sasaki, R.F. (1965). *The Zen koan: Its history and use in Rinzai Zen*. San Diego, CA: Harcourt Brace.

Montuori, A. (2005). Gregory Bateson and the challenge of transdisciplinarity. *Cybernetics and Human Knowing, 12*(1–2), 147–158.

Neill, J. & Kniskern, D. (Eds.). (1982). *From psyche to system: the evolving therapy of Carl Whitaker*. New York, NY: Guilford Press.

Pakman, M. (2004). On imagination: reconciling knowledge and life, or what does 'Gregory Bateson' stand for?, *Family Process, 43*(4), 413-23.

Pask, G. (1996). Heinz von Foerster's self-organisation, the progenitor of conversation and interaction theories. *Systems Research 13*(3), pp. 349-362.

Satir, V. (1988). *The new peoplemaking*. Palo Alto, CA: Science and Behavior Books, Inc.

Spencer-Brown, G. (1969). *Laws of form*. London, England: Allen & Unwin.

Stagoll, B. (2000). "Interactions Not Factions". In Dialogues of diversity in therapy: A virtual symposium, *Australian and New Zealand Journal of Marriage and Family Therapy, 21*(3), 124-126

Stephenson, H. & Keeney, B. (2011). Circular poetics and the "hypnosis of hypnosis", *The American Journal of Clinical Hypnosis, 54*(2), 86-88.

Suzuki, D. T. (1970). *The field of Zen: Contributions to the middle way, the journal of the Buddhist Society*. New York, NY: Harper & Row.

Suzuki, D. T. & Barrett, W. (1956). *Zen Buddhism: Selected writings of D. T. Suzuki*. Garden City, NY: Doubleday.

Suzuki, S. & Dixon, T. (2006) *Zen mind, beginner's mind*. Boston, MA: Shambhala Publications, Inc.

Thomas, F. N., Waits, R. A., & Hartsfield, G. L. (2007). The influence of Gregory Bateson: Legacy or vestige? *Kybernetes, 36*(7/8), 871–883.
Tyler, S. A, & Tyler, M.G. (1990). Foreword. In B.P. Keeney, *Improvisational therapy: A practical guide for creative clinical strategies* (pp. ix-xi). New York, NY: Guilford Press.
Varela, F. J. (1999). *Ethical know-how: Action, wisdom, and cognition.* Stanford, CA: Stanford University Press.
von Foerster, H. (Ed.). (1953). *Feedback mechanisms and circular causal systems in biology and the social sciences.* New York, NY: Josiah Macy, Jr. Foundation.
von Foerster, H. (1984). *Observing systems.* Salinas, CA: Intersystem Publications.
von Foerster, H. (1987). Cybernetics. In S.C. Shapiro (Ed.), *Encyclopedia for artificial intelligence* (Vol. 1, pp. 225-227). New York: Wiley.
von Foerster, H. (2003a). *Understanding understanding: Essays on cybernetics and cognition.* New York, NY: Springer-Verlag.
von Foerster, H. (2003b). Cybernetics of epistemology. In H. von Foerster (Ed.), *Understanding understanding: Essays on cybernetics and cognition* (pp. 229–246). New York, NY: Springer-Verlag.
von Foerster, H. (2003c). Ethics and second-order cybernetics. In H. von Foerster (Ed.), *Understanding understanding: Essays on cybernetics and cognition* (pp. 287–304). New York, NY: Springer-Verlag.
Watzlawick, P., Beavin, J., & Jackson, D. (1967). *Pragmatics of human communication: A study of interactional patterns, pathologies & paradoxes.* NY: W.W. Norton.
Watzlawick, P., Weakland, J. H., & Fisch, R. (1974). *Change: Principles of problem formation and problem resolution.* New York, NY: Norton.
Whitaker, C. (1976). Hindrance of theory clinical work. In P. Geurin (Ed.), *Family therapy: Theory and practice* (154-164). New York, NY: Gardner Press.
White, M. & Epston, D. (1990). *Narrative means to therapeutic ends.* New York, NY: W.W. Norton & Company.
Whitehead, A. N., & Russell, B. (1910). *Principia mathematica.* Cambridge, UK: Cambridge University Press.
Wordsworth, W. (1993). Preface to lyrical ballads. In M. H. Abrams (Ed.), *The Norton anthology of English literature, Vol. 2* (pp. 141–152). New York, NY: Norton. (Original work published 1800).
Yamada, K. (2004). *The gateless gate: The classic book of Zen koans.* Boston, MA: Wisdom.

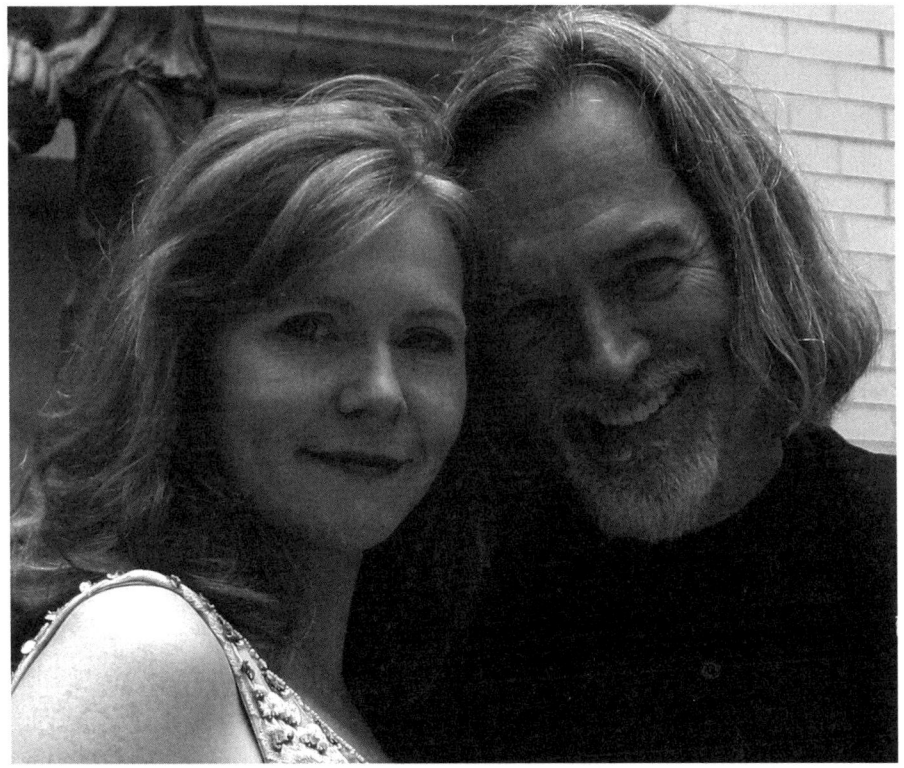

Photo by Frank Thomas

THE AUTHORS

HILLARY KEENEY, PH.D., spent over ten years working in the nonprofit sector as a leadership coach, diversity trainer, and community worker dedicated to youth leadership development and social justice. Hillary recently left the nonprofit sector to become a scholar and practitioner of creative approaches to personal and social change. She is presently Distinguished Visiting Professor in Psychology, Benemérita Universidad Autónoma de Puebla (BUAP), Mexico and Adjunct Faculty in the Creative Systemic Studies doctoral concentration at the University of Louisiana.

A seasoned trainer and dialogue facilitator, Hillary has co-written and facilitated over two hundred workshops and trainings ranging from postgraduate therapy education, creative coaching, diversity and racial justice issues, to collective organizational leadership. Hillary served as a diversity trainer with Allies for Change and spent three years with Public Allies training young leaders to do community change work in Los Angeles and Phoenix.

She received her B.A. in Women's Studies and Masters of Social Work from the University of Michigan. Her doctorate in Transformative Studies is from the California Institute for Integral Studies, San Francisco, and she has taught Gender, Women's, and Sexuality Studies at California State University. Hillary spent five years studying Zen Buddhism as a resident of the Zen Center of Los Angeles, and was awarded the Frederick P. Lenz Residential Fellowship for the Study of American Buddhism at Naropa University in Fall 2009.

Hillary has a true commitment to interdisciplinary scholarship and bringing contemporary people helping professions into greater relationship to the healing ways held inside great wisdom traditions. Hillary works with Bradford Keeney to provide postgraduate training to therapists and other mental health workers at conferences and workshops throughout the world including Mexico, Brazil, Australia, and Europe.

Her most recent books (co-authored with Bradford Keeney) include *A Arte de Beber Uma Taça de Amor* (Campinas, Brazil: IDPH Press, 2012), and *A Master Class in the Art of Performing Change* (Melbourne, Australia: PsychOz Publications, 2012).

BRADFORD KEENEY, PH.D., is an internationally renowned creative therapist, cybernetician, anthropologist of cultural healing traditions, and improvisational performer. He is presently Professor and Hanna Spyker Eminent Scholars Chair, University of Louisiana, Monroe, and has served as a professor, founder, and director of clinical doctoral programs in numerous universities. He is the originator of several orientations to psychotherapy including improvisational therapy, resource focused therapy, and creative therapy. A Fellow of the American Association for Marriage and Family Therapy, he received the Distinguished Lifetime Achievement Award from the Louisiana Association for Marriage and Family Therapy.

As a scholar, his classic text, *Aesthetics of Change,* was cited by Heinz von Foerster as one of the key texts of cybernetics, the original science of complexity. He is the inventor of recursive frame analysis, a research method that discerns patterns of transformation in conversation. As a fieldworker, Keeney has been called "the Marco Polo of psychology and an anthropologist of the spirit" by the editors of Utne Reader. He spent over a decade traveling the globe, living with spiritual teachers and healers who trusted him to share their words with others—modern cultures in need of elder wisdom. The result of Keeney's work is one of the broadest and most intense field studies of healing, chronicled in the critically acclaimed book series, *Profiles of Healing,* an eleven-volume encyclopedia of the world's healing practices.

Recognized as an ecstatic spiritual teacher and healer by numerous cultures, Keeney became a n/om-kxao (healer) with the Kalahari Bushmen. Megan Biesele, Ph.D., former member of the Harvard Kalahari Research Group, writes: "There is no question in the minds of the Bushman healers that Keeney's strength and purposes are coterminous with theirs. They affirmed his power as a healer." He is the subject of the book, *American Shaman: An Odyssey of Global Healing Traditions* written by psychologists Jeffrey Kottler and Jon Carlson, which won a Best Spiritual Book of 2005 award from *Spirituality & Health* magazine. A display honoring his breakthrough fieldwork and contributions to understanding the origin of human culture is permanently installed as an exhibition in the Origins Centre Museum, Johannesburg, South Africa.

Keeney has presented keynote addresses to professional audiences throughout the United States, Canada, Mexico, Europe, Africa, Japan, Central and South America, and Australia. He is the author of over 36 books including *The Bushman Way of Tracking God,* which won the prestigious Silver Nautilus national book award.

Their new website is
www.therapyheart.com